Praise for *Life Disrupted*

"Eloquent and funny. If you've experienced chronic illness, or if you care for someone who has, you need to read this book."
—Amy Tenderich, www.diabetesmine.com,
coauthor of *Know Your Numbers, Outlive Your Diabetes*

"As a person living with a chronic illness, it is inspiring to hear such a fresh and important voice. Laurie Edwards puts adversity in its place and teaches us to not only go on living, but to create a better life. High five, Sister!"
—Kris Carr, author of *Crazy, Sexy, Cancer*

"For those young people suffering from chronic illness, *Life Disrupted* offers strategy, advice, and hope. For those of us lucky enough to grow up without illness, it tells us how to be respectfully helpful to friends, family, and colleagues in this situation. Superb and engaging writing."
—Paul F. Levy, president and CEO of Beth Israel
Deaconess Medical Center, Boston,
www.runningahospital.blogspot.com

"A wise and valuable addition to the literature on chronic illness, illuminating with verve and wit the particular struggles faced by young adults. Ms. Edwards is a delightful and seasoned guide. She knows what the issues are, how to decipher them, and how to live a rich life while shuttling between hospitals and high heels."
—Dorothy Wall, author of *Encounters with the
Invisible: Unseen Illness, Controversy,
and Chronic Fatigue Syndrome*

"Laurie Edwards is a generous writer who describes with grace and clarity how she has learned to live with multiple chronic conditions. This book is a gift to young people who are navigating chronic illness, school, and their new adulthood all at once."
—Jessie Gruman, author of *AfterShock:
What to Do When the Doctor Gives You—
Or Someone You Love—a Devastating Diagnosis*

continued . . .

"Chronic illness needn't change your life for the worse if you let Laurie be your guide to everything from doctors to dating to why we sweat the small stuff (because sometimes that's all we feel we can control). Laurie Edwards is a compassionate confidante, an understanding friend, and a witty chronicler of all things chronic illness, even the not-so-pretty parts. Bravo!"
—Susan Milstrey Wells, author of *A Delicate Balance:
Living Successfully with Chronic Illness*

"Laurie Edwards is a life-enhancing writer. If you're a person with chronic illness, you should always keep this wonderful book handy." —Sarah M. Whitman, M.D., psychiatrist specializing in chronic pain management, www.howtocopewithpain.org

"Laurie Edwards has written a moving and meaningful description of the issues that people face when they live with unpredictable and debilitating disease. Her words reminded me of my own struggles—and her laughter helped me remember the good times, too." —Rosalind Joffe, author of *Women, Work, and Autoimmune Disease: Keep Working, Girlfriend!* and president of Chronic Illness Coach

"Both a practical and a philosophical guide for those navigating this heretofore uncharted territory."
—Lynn Royster, J.D., Ph.D., director of The Chronic Illness Initiative at The School for New Learning at DePaul University

"*Life Disrupted* is moving and often humorous, as Laurie Edwards informs readers about how they can navigate successfully through the medical storms, live well, and maintain fulfilling relationships." —Douglas Whynott, author of *Giant Bluefin* and *A Country Practice*

"The time for patient empowerment has come and Laurie Edwards' voice is leading the way. As a fellow lifelong patient, I appreciate her honesty in disclosing private patient moments which reflect the often unspoken truth of living with chronic illness." —Tiffany Christensen, www.sickgirlspeaks.com, author of *Sick Girl Speaks!: Lessons and Ponderings Along the Road to Acceptance*

LIFE DISRUPTED

LIFE DISRUPTED

Getting Real About Chronic Illness
in Your Twenties and Thirties

Laurie Edwards

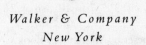

Walker & Company
New York

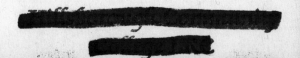

Published by Walker Publishing Company, Inc., New York
Distributed to the trade by Macmillan

All papers used by Walker & Company are natural, recyclable
products made from wood grown in well-managed forests. The
manufacturing processes conform to the environmental regulations
of the country of origin.

LIBRARY OF CONGRESS CATALOGING-IN-PUBLICATION DATA

Edwards, Laurie (Laurie Elizabeth)
Life disrupted : getting real about chronic illness in your twenties
and thirties / Laurie Edwards.—1st U.S. ed.
p. cm.
Includes bibliographical references.
ISBN-13: 978-0-8027-1649-1 (alk. paper)
ISBN-10: 0-8027-1649-0 (alk. paper)
1. Chronically ill. 2. Young adults—Diseases. I. Title.
RC108.E39 2008
618.92'0478—dc22
2008000245

Visit Walker & Company's Web site at www.walkerbooks.com

First U.S. edition 2008

1 3 5 7 9 10 8 6 4 2

Typeset by Westchester Book Group
Printed in the United States of America by Quebecor World Fairfield

*For Dorothy "Dollie" Shea, who loved books,
and John T. Shea Jr., who valued truth*

CONTENTS

INTRODUCTION

Y OUR CHART DOESN'T MENTION IT, but are you a nurse, by any chance? I mean, you know so much of the terminology," my nurse asked. Her name was Tracy, she looked like she was in her late twenties, a little older than me, and she brought into the stale hospital room a refreshing whiff of light perfume. I had never seen her among my batch of "regulars," but by the week's end she would know to bring diet ginger ale without being asked and would look aside when visitors arrived long after visiting hours ended.

We had just finished discussing my IV line and how I feared it was infiltrated and would likely need changing soon. It was July 2003, and I was in the hospital for the fifth time since the previous spring.

I chuckled slightly at her question, seeing that she was completely in earnest.

"No, I'm not a nurse . . . I'm a twenty-three-year patient," I said. "Seems like nursing may have been an easier way to get so informed, huh?" I asked, using my free arm to motion to the oxygen tubes and the heart monitor banked to my left, obvious indicators of my lifelong experience with illness.

It wasn't the first time I'd been asked if I were a medical professional and it wouldn't be the last, but it would be the first time that I stopped to consider the implications of Tracy's assumptions, and the value of my patient experience. In fact, later that same summer it was this recognition that prompted me to leave my doctor and hospital and embark on the diagnostic journey that finally yielded the correct diagnoses I'd waited a lifetime to get. I have primary ciliary dyskinesia (PCD), a rare genetic respiratory disorder that means the cilia (tiny structures) that normally line the lungs and respiratory tract and help clear out mucus and infection either do not work or are not there at all. The symptoms of PCD—frequent infections, thick mucus, decreased oxygenation, etc.—are similar to those of cystic fibrosis (CF), as are the treatments. According to the PCD Foundation, there are only about a thousand documented cases of PCD in the entire United States, though an estimated twenty-five thousand people may have the condition but have yet to be accurately diagnosed. Because I have several other medical conditions (bronchiectasis, celiac disease, and thyroid disease, to name but a few), it was often difficult to tease out where one disease ended and another began, so I have spent most of my life looking for explanations of my illness that match my *experience* of illness.

The stories in this book stretch across the younger adult age and disease spectrum, from Jade Cooper, a twenty-year-old college student living with chronic pancreatitis, to Jenni Prokopy, a thirty-four-year-old fibromyalgia patient-cum-advocate. Among others, you'll also hear from thirty-three-year-old Vicki Klein, a cystic fibrosis patient who is on the lung transplant list and the mother of a toddler son; Kerri Morrone, a twenty-eight-year-old type 1 diabetic who is a columnist and diabetes blogger, and Angela Ayoub, a twenty-three-year-old college student living with Ehlers-Danlos syndrome, a rare connective tissue disease that affects skin, joints, and the vascular system. Brian Sercus, a twenty-five-year-old CF patient, adds a much-needed male voice to this discussion on chronic illness. And then there is me, the storyteller, the daughter of two chronically ill parents and the sister of two healthy older brothers whose lives have all been impacted by my mélange of conditions over the years.

Like the greater patient population our experiences represent, our conditions range from the life-altering to the life-threatening, from autoimmune diseases to genetic disorders, from those that require daily vigilance to those that flare periodically. Some of them are rare, others affect millions; some we were born with, others emerged later in life. Yet all these differences speak to even more compelling commonalities: these conditions are treatable, not curable, a distinction that is more important in today's health care system than ever before, and these conditions in some way complicate the already complex terrain that people in their twenties and thirties must navigate. Our responses and adaptations to illness are as different as our physical symptoms and treatment plans are, but universal themes of acceptance, identity, and survival are independent of disease category and pathology.

Illness can be isolating, but through research and interviews with other patients, I found that I was not alone in my quest to balance the competing desires of my body and my spirit. For one thing, better technology and advanced treatment mean people with serious childhood illnesses are living into adulthood in larger numbers than ever before. Combined with the millions of people who are diagnosed with chronic diseases in their twenties and thirties, it's clear that the population of young adults who are trying to forge productive, dynamic lives while contending with bodies that do not always behave as we'd like them to is enormous. Never before have medicine and society had to contend with issues like the effects of caregiving on young marriages and relationships or seriously ill young adults having children on such a large scale, but here we are.

So where do we go now?

I realized after my conversation with my nurse Tracy that July day in 2003 that I *was* an expert, whether or not I even want this distinction. I haven't gone to medical school and I've never received training as a nurse, but I have something even more valuable: a lifetime of experience. I have all the accoutrements to show for it: proficiency with medical jargon, a hefty medical file, numerous surgeries, and a daunting list of diagnoses. But more important, in addition to scar tissue and invoices, I've also collected a lot of hard-earned knowledge about how to live with chronic illness. Sure, I know the frustration of a prolonged hospitalization or an incorrect diagnosis, but I also know how many martinis I can consume when I go out before they interfere with my medications, and how to plan a swanky New Year's Eve party from my sickbed. I've seen all ends of the medical spectrum, from the major near-death experiences in the ICU to the minor indignities of trying to kiss my then-boyfriend with a GI tube taped to my cheek and snaked down my nose into my stomach.

The power of the patient experience is the impetus of this book. From navigating the institution of medicine to dealing with illness in the public sphere to the influence of illness on personal relationships, the three sections in this book depend on the expertise of patients to stake their claims. In a sense, the parts follow the natural trajectory of the chronically ill patient, who first receives a diagnosis in an office or hospital, travels through the public domain of work or school, and then returns home, where he or she must confront the impact of illness on family and friends. As a twenty-seven-year-old patient with multiple chronic illnesses who is also a writer, college instructor, wife, daughter, aunt, and friend, I've seen over and over the many ways illness can infiltrate these other roles. I am not interested in exploring the word "healthy" in this book, a term so slippery and so nuanced it practically has no meaning to me. What matters to me are terms like "well" and "health*ier*" since they speak to the real truth of chronic illness. Being well means being able to find a place for chronic illness within the context of our relationships and our professional lives, not at the expense of them.

PART 1

Medical Life: On Doctors, Hospitals,
and the Nature of Expertise

1.

ILLNESS VERSUS DISEASE—
IT'S MORE THAN JUST WORDS

*The patient narrative is an essential
piece of the patient experience*

WHETHER YOU'RE A LIFELONG PATIENT seeing yet
another new specialist or someone new to the exam
room, you face the same decisions in that moment when
you begin to tell your story to the doctor: *Where do I start?
Which details should I include? Can I make this person understand how I feel, what my life is like?*

Maybe you're distracted by the cold table or the annoying
rustle and crinkle of the paper sheet underneath you, or perhaps you're worried about making a positive first impression
so you smooth your hair or sit up a bit straighter when the
doctor enters the room. Maybe you're anxious about a potential diagnosis, or hopeful about a new medication. You
may have even brought a list of items to discuss with your
physician, symptoms or observations you don't want to forget to mention but fear you might. Either way, the dialogue

between patient and physician depends on each person dispensing facts and interpreting situations. In this sense, the exchange rooted in science and fact is profoundly human.

Before we can even begin to navigate the intricacies of the health care system, we should first understand how our individual medical histories and prior relationships with medical professionals shape and define the very system of which we're all a part. The forms and charts, the requisition slips and insurance waivers, the discharge notes and prescription pads—all these interactions and communications that eventually involve so many other people in our lives begin and end with one patient in an exam room discussing his or her health and a physician making notes and piecing together initial impressions of symptoms.

Without this interaction, where the patient's history becomes the physician's compass, the rest of organized medicine cannot exist. Pretty obvious, right? It's tempting to think so. But consider the idea that physicians are trained to recognize, diagnose, and, when possible, cure, or at least treat, disease. Disease, then, is the stuff of laboratories, specimens, and procedures—the result of diagnostic inquiries and tests, the ruling out of one thing by the presence of another. *Illness*, though, refers to the actual experience of living with conditions, and unlike the language of disease, this is a vocabulary that belongs to the patient. Rather than numbers or quantities, it concerns emotions and perceptions. For example, I tell my doctor about the tightness in my chest, the congested cough that keeps me up at night, the waves of tiredness that creep up on me suddenly. When I do, my illness is a pattern of infections and complications that is a part of everyday life. My disease is something different, something defined not by my descriptions or anecdotes, but by numbers: oxygen saturation, pulmonary function tests, sputum specimens. For the migraine sufferer discussing potential triggers, the diabetic worrying about uncontrolled blood sugars, and the arthritic explaining an especially severe pain flare, the tension between what we feel and how those physical and emotional feelings translate into the language of medicine is the same.

In *Illness and Culture in the Postmodern Age*, David B. Morris highlights the fundamental difference between the two: "The power to make us sick or well inheres not only in microbes or medications but in images and stories . . . the main assumption underlying the distinction between disease and illness is that knowledge falls into two broad categories, objective and subjective."[1] Morris goes on to argue that in today's postmodern world the patient experience cannot be boiled down into such simple terms as either purely subjective or objective, and he's correct—thankfully. The once limited dialogue between patient and practitioner, between subjective experience and objective knowledge, has shifted. Comprehensive Internet health sites, patient forums and interactive discussion boards, health blogs, and interviews yield unprecedented ways for patients to be active participants in the health care system. We can type our symptoms into a search engine and explore the results; we can join online health communities and social networking sites and debate the merits of certain medications over others; we can e-mail our physicians and nurse practitioners and ask about refilling a prescription or discuss a side effect. The more patients and health care providers communicate and the more commonalities our modes of language share, the closer we get to more accurate diagnoses and more effective treatment plans.

Every patient is a storyteller responsible for narrating the particular details of his or her unique history. We weed through aches and pains, side effects and complications, and pick the details that best serve the purpose of our particular story. But it doesn't end there. At the other end of the story is the physician who is hearing it, someone whose own perspective allows him or her to gravitate toward certain facts over others, whose mind wraps around some images and descriptions more than others. In that way, physicians and patients actually share many qualities—when faced with a barrage of signals and information, we each do our very best to filter out the most essential chunks and use them to make decisions. I believe in the strength of telling our individual stories, of actively participating in a system that can seem anonymous and overwhelming. Only when we offer up our experiences and subject them to the interpretation of clinicians can the dialogue that is so essential to our health begin.

2.

EXPERT DIAGNOSIS

*Diagnosis depends on listening to
your body and finding physicians
willing to do the same*

I HAVE ALWAYS BEEN what doctors called "an enigma."
They said this to me while leaning back in their swivel
chairs, peering over my lab reports. They said this to me
when prescribing antibiotics for rare bacterial infections,
wondering how I contracted them. They said this to me
while ordering tests and oxygen in the ER, and asked me if
they have seen me before, they're sure they have seen me
before. Of course they have, it was last Thanksgiving or
early May or that Christmas two years ago, they suddenly
remembered with a sheepish smile.

So how did I get from medical mystery to someone whose
labels actually matched her experiences? The first step in the
process was that I began to truly listen to what my body was
telling me instead of listening to what the doctors thought
they heard, a distinction so critical that everything else about

diagnosis and doctor relationships depends on it. Symptoms are symptoms regardless of their classification, so it is not as if receiving a diagnosis magically confers on you the designation of "sick." Certainly my experience of not being able to breathe was every bit as real and visceral when I didn't have the labels of PCD or bronchiectasis; it was my quality of life that changed. Diagnosis divides your perspective into "before" and "after" in terms of clarity and understanding. How can you begin to integrate the realities and treatments of your condition and feel better if you don't know what it is?

For some patients, diagnosis itself can be fairly clear-cut. Once Kerri Morrone began feeling feverish and increasingly sluggish, it didn't take too much time for her physician to diagnose the then six-year-old with type 1 diabetes. Similarly, like the majority of cystic fibrosis patients, Vicki Klein and Brian Sercus tested positive for the disorder at a very young age, so it was always clear to their families and their physicians what was wrong. Despite how serious or unwelcome the news is, for diseases with very clear tests, at least the diagnostic process itself is conclusive.

Except we don't always get such concrete answers. There are a lot of factors that can account for this, all of which will be explored in further detail throughout the book. For one, many types of chronic illness have symptoms like fatigue, joint pain, gastrointestinal distress, or muscle weakness that readily overlap with symptoms of other conditions, making it difficult to isolate the primary cause. Certain chronic conditions—fibromyalgia (FM), lupus, and chronic fatigue syndrome (CFS), for example—have no one definitive diagnostic test or indicator, meaning physicians often have to rely on clinical observations, patient history, and reported symptoms that share similarities with established benchmark criteria to hazard a diagnosis.

Jenni Prokopy's quest to figure out what was wrong with her follows a trajectory that is, unfortunately, all too familiar for many patients with chronic illness. Her health history included frequent childhood infections, ear tubes, viral meningitis at thirteen, and mononucleosis during high school. The chronic pain in her limbs was dismissed as "growing pains" and no one made the connection between those pains and all the other signs of illness that manifested themselves throughout her life. She was twenty-five when she was diagnosed with asthma, anxiety, Raynaud's phenomenon (an autoimmune disorder that primarily affects the blood vessels in the fingers and toes), and fibromyalgia.

"The process of diagnosis was awful. It was pretty typical of fibromyalgia and chronic fatigue syndrome—all kinds of exams and appointments and CT scans," she says. When she was diagnosed almost ten years ago, awareness and understanding of FM and CFS was nascent; people still referred to chronic fatigue as "yuppie fever" then and even those practitioners who identified the conditions in their patients didn't always have helpful strategies for living with them. Jenni felt that some doctors didn't believe what she was saying, and the first doctor who actually looked at her symptoms and history of chronic pain and diagnosed her with fibromyalgia told her to "get used to a life of pain." She offered her Advil and a pamphlet about the disease and sent her on her way.

The support group for FM patients she joined shortly after her diagnosis increased her sense of frustration. It was filled with people years older who told her things like, "You're too young to be sick" or "It can't be *that* bad, you're so young!" Despite the fact that many autoimmune disorders and chronic illnesses emerge during childbearing years, such attitudes about illness and age are not uncommon, and they make this journey more complicated. It also compounds the isolating nature of illness—not only are you sidetracked from the majority of your healthy peers by illness, but also you're further marginalized from the very patient group you can finally claim as your own.

Jenni struggled with the decision to get a second opinion; she felt her role as patient meant doing what the doctors said and following their treatment plans without comment. "Patients have to really step up and take a lot more responsibility for managing their care than we sometimes want to," she says. Now Jenni is an outspoken advocate, embodying this idea of responsibility and proactive approaches to self-care. Her Web site, ChronicBabe.com, is specifically designed to cater to young women living with chronic illnesses. Her change in attitude came once she decided to squelch her doubts and push for the appropriate diagnosis and resources, knowing that her chronic pain was not something she should ignore. As a result, her current treatment plan calls for much more than Advil; for example, she exercises, stretches, and has utilized biofeedback and changes in diet and lifestyle to help minimize her pain.

Jade Cooper's experience in receiving a diagnosis for the terrible stomach and back pain she has experienced since the fifth grade was as frustrating as Jenni's, and in Jade's case, age was even more of a complicating factor. Throughout her adolescence, her pain was dismissed by doctors who said it was the result of stress. Jade describes chronic pancreatitis as being similar to cirrhosis of the liver, except that the organ affected is the pancreas—and the pancreas can't rejuvenate itself. Though gallstones and heredity can also cause it, chronic pancreatitis is most common among older alcoholics. As such, it certainly wasn't an obvious affliction for a teenage girl to have. On top of that, parents and doctors view adolescence as a particularly turbulent and stressful time, so attributing Jade's searing pain to stress, especially when she didn't appear to have any of the more common maladies that would cause such pain, seemed reasonable to her physician and her family at the time.

"My parents had never dealt with illness before. They didn't know any better than to trust the doctors," Jade says—and of course, neither did she. It wasn't until she was a freshman in college and showed up at the urgent care facility in the most excruciating pain of her life that she found doctors who were willing to go through a lot of trial and error to find the cause of her symptoms. Her freshman year was filled with hospitalizations and surgery as well as challenges to manage her pain, but she finally knew what was wrong with her, and with that knowledge, she could move forward, leaving the stress label behind her.

"My parents had a steep learning curve. They felt really bad for trusting the doctors all that time. I *knew* it wasn't just stress, but you just don't know not to trust what the doctor tells you," she says. For adolescent patients making the transition from being under their parents' care to controlling their own disease management, this issue of patient authority is particularly complex. Jade knew her parents were thinking and acting in her best interest, but she also knew her body was telling her something very different from what the doctors had convinced her parents was wrong. Fortunately, she found the right physician at the right time in her life—as a college freshman with burgeoning independence—to exert more control over both her diagnosis and her prognosis.

Clearly this hesitancy to question the conclusions made by physicians pervades any discussion of misdiagnosis. But as Jade's story illustrates, diagnosing unusual conditions is also confounded by the fact that physicians aren't used to seeing them in their patient populations. Doctors may not recognize the symptoms for what they are or, as in Jade's case, may assume they are caused by more common conditions. In *How Doctors Think*, Dr. Jerome Groopman writes, "Experts studying misguided care have recently concluded that the majority of errors are due to flaws in physician thinking, not technical mistakes. In one study of misdiagnoses that caused serious harm to patients, some 80 percent could be accounted for by a cascade of cognitive errors."[1] Such errors are not intentional or malicious but are the result of a system that relies on algorithms and decision trees—if a common symptom presents itself, then the most common cause is the first one considered, and often the one assigned to the patient. Herein Groopman emphasizes an especially relevant point: "Clinical algorithms can be useful for run-of-the-mill diagnosis and treatment . . . But they quickly fall apart when a doctor needs to think outside their boxes, when symptoms are vague, or multiple and confusing, or when test results are inexact."[2]

These ideas resonate with me deeply since they speak to the same conundrum my father faced when he was just about the age I am now. His high fevers, severe muscle weakness, and other lab results initially pointed toward the more common diagnosis of muscular dystrophy. After languishing for seven years while being treated for the wrong disease, he was correctly diagnosed with polymyositis, an extremely rare neuromuscular disease. In the years of misdiagnosis, a seven-pound tumor, likely associated with his polymyositis, slowly ravaged his kidney and was only identified when he began hemorrhaging and nearly died. Doctors removed his kidney and pronounced him diabetic from the steroids he took for the muscular dystrophy he never had, but at last he finally had the right diagnosis.

Clearly I don't fall far from my family tree in regard to

dubious diagnoses. I'd been sick literally since birth, and for many years we didn't even realize I had the wrong diagnosis. We did know I had an IgG immune deficiency that left me prone to infections; I had multiple ear, nose, and throat surgeries every year and spent weeks in isolation in the hospital with resistant infections. Blood and pus would stream from my ears, and I once had my head cut open to drain an infection that was encroaching on my brain. Aside from the steady stream of surgeries, the main constant in my life was the struggle to breathe. I'd been diagnosed with asthma as a toddler, and by first grade I had two different kinds of nebulizers at home and still needed to go to the hospital frequently. I developed bronchitis at least five times a year and was always wheezing and coughing up gunk. I carried my inhalers with me everywhere, and like a lot of asthmatic children, I often had to bring notes to gym class and missed social events because of my cough or my wheeze. I was always on steroids. *Always*.

The older I got, the worse my respiratory problems became. By college, I was spending weeks at a time as an inpatient. I would cough for hours and hours at a time, cough until my throat was hoarse and raw and my ribs were sore, and the phlegm never went away, no matter how much I coughed up. I heard phrases like "exacerbations of unknown origin" and "atypical asthma resistant to treatment" thrown around by my pulmonary team, and it didn't escape my notice that the sicker I got, the more personally they seemed to take it. It didn't make any sense; steroids should reduce inflammation, and inflammation was the main cause of symptoms in asthma. So why weren't the toxic doses of steroids that destroyed my metabolism, rendered my bones as brittle as twigs, and eventually shut down my adrenal system working?

It wasn't until I graduated from Georgetown University and moved from Washington, D.C., back to my hometown of Boston and proceeded to spend even more time in the hospital that I reached my breaking point. If the drugs that destroyed so many other parts of my body weren't even helping, maybe we weren't treating the right condition. I pointed to the ever-full cup of phlegm at my bedside as evidence that something other than asthma had to be causing it. "Have you ever known asthma to produce this much phlegm?" I asked an intern, flushed with indignation. It was a sweltering summer day in 2003 and I lay in the ICU coughing up yet more phlegm. She shook her head no.

It was that intern's subtle but definitive shake of the head, along with my nurse Tracy's remark, that finally snapped me into action. I was determined to find an answer that made sense instead of the worn, tired explanations I'd heard for years. My parents and I researched the top airway disorder specialists from my hospital bed—I always bring my computer to the hospital as part of my survival gear—and one of them agreed to see me as soon as I was discharged. That first appointment set up the chain of events, tests, and procedures that eventually led me to the diagnoses of PCD and bronchiectasis and enabled me to adopt a very different course of treatment.

When I look back, I can see why the asthma diagnosis was, at first, a reasonable one. Twenty years ago, I'm not even sure the technology to identify and diagnose PCD existed, and even if it had, it didn't mean my pediatrician would have ever heard of it, never mind recognized it. A toddler wheezes and coughs and gets sick a lot, and she tests negative for the CF sweat test; so the most common and likely diagnosis is asthma. For millions of children out there, that diagnosis *is* correct, and the steps in that decision-making process are logical. But it only fit me on the surface, and it failed to encompass all the other pieces that formed my composite picture. For example, trademark signs of PCD—premature birth with collapsed lungs, frequent ear and sinus infections, recurrent respiratory infections, thick mucus that doesn't clear, underlying immune deficiency disorders, to name a few—were always present in my life. Muddled by the asthma diagnosis, these competing facts didn't have a chance to get full consideration. Once I was labeled an asthmatic, then every flare, infection, and exacerbation was pathologized and treated from that singular perspective.

Doctor-patient relationships are an indispensable part of a successful diagnostic journey, and both the relationship and the eventual diagnosis itself depend on compatibility and communication. Like a first date with someone, the first appointment with a physician tells so much: Does the doctor look you in the eye when you tell your history? Does she ask probing follow-up questions that show she understands the connections you are beginning to draw? These subtle cues reveal so much.

There is a distinct, critical difference between hearing and listening, and you can tell within seconds which a new physician, specialist, or consultant is doing. When they hear, they merely look for confirmation of what they have already decided, as evidenced by my asthma label. When they listen, however, they integrate the patient's perspective on his or her body with their clinical one. This distinction was the litmus test I used when I needed to find a specialist who was familiar with PCD and bronchiectasis. I scoured the Web profiles of doctors my insurance company listed as "in network," paying close attention to patient satisfaction evaluations. I checked with neighbors who were doctors and spread names out among my contacts, scrutinizing the way people described the doctors they knew. What I was interested in hearing about was personality and bedside manner. If those characteristics were the first things that came to people's minds when I asked them about a particular doctor, that said a lot about what he or she would be like as my doctor.

After all this reconnaissance—and of course I Googled him too—there was a new man in my life, Dr. Bruce Levy. What did it do for me? He looked me in the eyes the entire time we met. He shook my hand when he entered, and he asked insightful questions that proved to me he wasn't just skimming my files and nodding along, that he had pored over my case file and cared about making this first appointment a productive one. This immediately made me more relaxed and comfortable disclosing my medical history. A doctor doesn't—or shouldn't—view what we say as a laundry list of complaints but as necessary tools to guide him or her toward better treatment. The more we disclose, the more both parties benefit.

With Dr. Levy, our relationship was sealed during our second appointment, when he told me we'd go over all my blood and lab work in a minute and then discuss treatment options, but first he wanted to hear what was new with me. How was my schoolwork going? Was I enjoying teaching? And did I have any new writing projects in the works?

He remembered, I thought. He really had been listening.

Stories like Jenni's, Jade's, and mine echo the experiences of millions of patients. My intention here is not to pit the medical education of doctors against the experiential education of patients but rather to draw the greatest strengths from each. Like many who have endured long journeys toward diagnosis, I have an entire lifetime of training. It was only when I had the confidence to act on the repeated signals my body gave me and reject a label I knew intrinsically did not fit me that I was able to find the people with the right answers and we could work together.

3.

HUNCHES THAT HEAL

*The importance of embracing
instinct goes both ways*

I F LISTENING AND INTERACTING is one component of the doctor-patient dynamic and the diagnostic process, then instinct is the other. It's pretty clear by now that, as patients, it is so important that we listen to our bodies and pursue alternative routes of diagnosis and treatment when the standard course of action isn't working. But what can get overshadowed is the fact that it is equally critical for physicians to embrace their instincts too. Medicine is dictated by science, yet to answer the most elusive questions, doctors sometimes need to be willing to put instinct first and let the science follow.

"It just hit me the other day, the possibility of celiac disease. I can't explain it. I was at my desk last week, and out of nowhere, you popped into mind, and I thought, 'She's celiac, I know it,'" my rheumatologist said. She drew my blood as she spoke (she's the only doctor I have who personally draws the blood), looking for initial evidence of celiac disease. Celiac disease is an autoimmune disorder in which the body cannot tolerate gluten, a protein found in wheat, barley, rye, and many other grains. Left unchecked, celiac disease slowly destroys the small intestine and can cause serious complications, but if the celiac adheres to a strict gluten-free diet, then that damage will be virtually eliminated and all other symptoms will be kept at bay.

"You have no idea how many patients come to me with all sorts of bizarre symptoms and it turns out to be celiac disease. I'm only surprised I didn't think of it before. With your family history, it makes so much sense," she said, knowing that there is a strong genetic component to celiac disease and that my uncle has it. In addition, autoimmune disorders are triggered by an immune response in which the body begins to mistakenly attack its own components, including its joints, muscles, and tissues. These faulty responses, in turn, trigger more immune reactions, so patients often have more than one autoimmune disorder. Along with my uncle's celiac disease, my family history includes my mother's severe rheumatoid arthritis and my father's polymyositis, so it is not surprising that an autoimmune disorder like celiac disease would manifest itself in me.

I had started seeing this doctor for arthritis flares in my lower back when I was in sixth grade, and though they have since subsided, I've continued seeing her into adulthood for tendonitis in my hips and arms, chronic fatigue, and joint pain associated with withdrawal from steroids, among other things. This fateful appointment came in mid-December 2003, the same time I was working toward my final respiratory diagnoses, a process she watched with a mix of compassion and indignation. "Specialists who are used to being right enjoy a challenge. You're a challenge. So they put you in their carefully constructed diagnostic boxes, sure they will be right. When you do not fit inside their box, they are not willing to build a new one, because that would mean admitting their error. And, Laurie, don't forget something," she said, pushing her stylish black rectangular glasses up on her nose and peering at me with intense blue eyes. "You're not simply a medical challenge. You keep them on their toes. You've been around the block too many times to just be a yes-person."

What draws me to her, what sustains me through the long hours spent in her waiting room, the traffic congestion on the commute to her suburban office, is the fact the she is no yes-person either. She's willing to take risks and to act on impulse on occasion. I take delight in the fact that, more often than not, she can piece together what is wrong with me more quickly and efficiently than anyone else by following her instinct. With that initial blood test in her office, I was on my way to piecing together the final missing element in my health history.

I can't blame my rheumatologist for not automatically spotting celiac disease in the midst of so much of my medical clutter. Like many autoimmune disorders, celiac disease is hard to identify because the symptoms so often look like many other things. There is no "typical" constellation of symptoms, and many people with the disorder do not present with more obvious signs like gastrointestinal problems or weight loss due to inadequate nutrient absorption. Like me, some experience fatigue and muscle pain as major complaints. Other celiacs exhibit no external symptoms at all. For these reasons, not only is celiac disease one of the most prevalent autoimmune disorders, but it is also one of the most underdiagnosed. According to the Celiac Sprue Association, an estimated 1 out of 133 people have it, yet only 3 percent of these people know it, meaning a staggering 2.1 million people suffer from it but lack a diagnosis.[1]

The process of adopting a gluten-free (GF) lifestyle—and I say "lifestyle" because, as with diabetes, adhering to the protocol is so much more than simply being on a restricted diet—is something that will be explored in later chapters, but the immediate benefits of this huge transition were obvious and indisputable. Within one month of eliminating all gluten from my diet—good-bye pita bread, bagels, soy sauce, cream of wheat—my sinuses were clear for the first time in my life (an unexpected boon, since no one had attributed my sinus congestion to anything but my lung and immune deficiency diseases), I had dropped eleven pounds, I had more energy, and most convincingly, my blood work and other tests now looked normal. Since I'd had hundreds of sinus headaches and undergone surgeries to drain my sinuses, I was willing to embrace the GF lifestyle forever based on my sinus relief alone, never mind that my persistent joint pain was less severe and my exhaustion diminished. The fact that going gluten-free repaired my small intestines and generally meant I was a healthier person whose autoimmune system was no longer completely haywire were added perks.

To this day, my doctor can't explain what made her think of celiac disease that December day, what line of thought or inquiry sparked her intuition and made her call me and have me come in right away, but I am grateful for whatever it was. I no longer had graham crackers mixed into my frozen yogurt or the ability to be in any way unconscious in my food choices, but I had that missing piece in the diagnostic disaster that was my medical history—and I had instinct, our mutual emerging ally, to thank for it.

4.

THE RIGHT TO REFUSE

*Voicing dissent doesn't make you a
difficult patient—it makes you an
empowered one*

W HILE WE USUALLY DESIRE to be "good patients"—
to appear diligent and committed to improving our
health, to be docile and gracious—that sense of diligence
and accommodation can become blind obedience, something far more troubling. This happens the moment we forget that, as patients, we still have the right to say no.

Since I was more familiar with my endocrine, respiratory, and autoimmune systems than anyone, I usually knew
when to question the experts. In fact, this questioning is
what led to my finally receiving the correct diagnoses. As a
result, I had more knowledge than ever before, and because
of that, I had power. I spent a lot of time undergoing procedures and shuffling from one office to the next with my new
medical team, but I knew *why* I was doing it. When I got
conflicting opinions about what turned out to be an adrenal

disorder, I had the confidence to leave one hospital and seek the appropriate treatment elsewhere.

Recently I encountered a problem that forced me to leave my comfort zone and resulted in my temporary reversion to being a submissive patient. I went to see a fertility specialist because my husband, John, and I knew that people with PCD are often infertile and we wanted to get as much information as we could to plan for our future. All my years of medical problems, surgeries, and tests never included any of the terms that suddenly became so important, and any confidence or authority I thought I had quickly disintegrated. It was like I was a new patient. I had peripheral knowledge of terms like in vitro fertilization and surrogacy, but I knew the facts and information in a general sense. It was a whole different situation when someone was using those terms in reference to my body and my reproductive potential. Suddenly I wasn't an expert anymore, so I clung to the only role available to me, one that was comforting in its familiarity: that of the good patient. The word "no" flew out of my lexicon altogether. I didn't ask for clarifications or explanations, even though my mind raced with questions.

I left my brief consult with a daunting list of blood tests and procedures to rule out other, unrelated fertility problems and the names of other subspecialists I needed to visit. I set about scheduling follow-up appointments and consultations, matching my pacing to that of the well-intentioned doctor even though I felt rushed and overwhelmed.

I was on patient autopilot.

I needed to book a particularly invasive and painful procedure, one that would rule out a condition my fertility specialist didn't think I had but still wanted to confirm. It was a game of diagnostic exclusion I'd played for years. I went back and forth with the busy practice for two weeks, and used up far too many of my daytime cell phone minutes on hold. I considered all the time I'd devoted to exams and physical therapy and consults and procedures and surgeries over the years. I thought about all the things I hadn't been able to do because I was too busy catering to my health. Right now, I wasn't willing to trade more time and inflict more pain for the purposes of ruling out an unlikely diagnosis. I'd get around to it, certainly, but not at the expense of so much else.

"Her job is to lay out your options and her recommendations. Your job is to decide which of those is right for you," a friend pointed out to me.

Of course my friend was right, but the issue of patient authority is never that concrete. At thirty-three, Vicki is a longtime veteran of cystic fibrosis, someone who is also informed about and diligent toward her health. Like me, she is all too aware of this deeply ingrained archetype of the "good patient." However, Vicki has rarely made the mistake of letting her own authority as a patient get overwhelmed by a tangle of facts and figures and misplaced deference. "To be perfectly candid, I am not what doctors call an 'ideal patient,'" she confesses. This isn't to say she is noncompliant—in fact, she is meticulous about her medical regimen and never, *never* misses a chest physiotherapy session, a nebulizer treatment, or a doctor's appointment. However, she fears she's earned the label of "difficult patient" because she regularly questions her physicians and challenges procedures. This tendency is more pronounced when she undergoes hospitalizations, which are particularly emotional periods for her. The more she feels the loss of control that being in the hospital causes, the more likely she is to exert her opinions and confront authority.

She imagines her doctors saying to themselves, "God,

every little battle she has to fight," and though she is some-what sheepish about this and wants to work on it, she doesn't apologize for being her own advocate. For instance, when she is in the hospital, she is adamant about not allow-ing her vital signs to be taken after eleven P.M. and before seven A.M. so she can rest. Cystic fibrosis patients aren't of-ten hospitalized for acute emergencies; more likely, routine maintenance techniques like IV flushes to combat infections are what bring Vicki to the hospital. She doesn't see a need to disrupt her sleep for vitals to be taken or blood drawn in the middle of the night and will say no as many times as it takes for the night staff to comply. These are the types of demands she won't back down from simply because that's the way things are usually done.

Thinking back to my friend's point, it's clear that's exactly what Vicki is doing in these moments—sorting through the recommended course of action and dismissing those steps that are not in her best interest as a patient. At its core, Vicki's story points to the need for balance between these competing interests: protecting your body and your auton-omy while at the same time assimilating into an institution that is overwhelming in its rules, standards, and hierarchy.

While Vicki self-identifies as someone who occasionally takes the proactive approach too far, certainly the opposite tack is just as problematic and far more prevalent. In de-scribing the events surrounding her fibromyalgia diagnosis, Jenni also identifies this tension between what constitutes a proactive patient and a difficult one. When doctors didn't believe what she was telling them, her initial reaction was to temper her complaints and hold back from questioning their opinions. "I didn't want to be a hypochondriac," she says. There it is, laid bare, that niggling worry that so many chronically ill patients have experienced—we don't want to come off as whiny or intractable. In our sickest moments we need medicine far more than it needs us, and challenging that institution when we're most vulnerable can be extremely difficult.

Jenni eventually exercised her own authority as a patient. She dismissed the very same doctors who dismissed her symptoms, mustering the confidence to say no to a line of thinking that wasn't helpful or healthful. Perhaps that should be the way we really define what a good patient is— an empowered one.

5.

ASSUMPTIONS ARE A MUTUAL AFFLICTION

There is such a thing as being too
confident in our knowledge as
patients

JUST AS PHYSICIANS can sometimes make assumptions that aren't always conducive to accurate diagnoses or treatments, we experienced patients can at times rely on our previous education too much. It isn't a question of being blasé but of becoming so acclimated to being chronic patients that we don't always see warning signs for what they are. Most of the time, confidence is a huge asset for patients and allows us to be our own best advocates. But there is a downside to such confidence—on occasion, it has lulled me into thinking I was inviolable, when I'm clearly not. I've learned the hard way that there is actually some benefit to the "new patient" experience, that sometimes allowing ourselves to feel scared or overwhelmed is exactly what we *should* be doing.

The most striking example of this occurred during my sophomore year in college, when I'd been sick for weeks with bronchitis that didn't respond to antibiotics. Things got so bad that I couldn't inhale without coughing and I had a stabbing, piercing pain in my chest every time I inhaled. This is the point when most people would consider seeking additional medical attention, but I was busy with end-of-semester activities and figured the extra symptoms were related to the change in the weather. Had I not been so quick to dismiss my body's signals and assume I knew what was going on, perhaps I would have sought medical treatment before developing pneumonia and having a partially collapsed lung, which required being rushed to the hospital and put in the trauma room where the sign on the door read RESUSCITATION TEAM MEMBERS ONLY.

Fantastic call on my part, no?

The line between adapting to physical problems and ignoring them is precariously thin. Again, I believe a lot of this has to do with the innate nature of chronic disease—our symptoms may ebb and flow, but they will never go away completely, so we have to learn to get by in spite of them. At the same time, if we become too immune to physical complaints, we risk putting our health in jeopardy. Angela Ayoub, who has Ehlers-Danlos syndrome, has had to learn to tolerate the chronic, severe discomfort that accompanies her disease. Since her dislocations and sprains are frequent and she leads a busy life as a full-time student and a full-time employee, she's adapted to needing to pop her joints back into place and the constant disruption this entails. She doesn't get scared or alarmed when, for example, her shoulder dislocates. She knows exactly why it's happening and exactly what needs to be done to fix it, and she tries to ignore the searing pain as much as possible.

For the most part, Angela's approach is effective, since it means she continues to accomplish her goals and lead as normal a life as possible. Yet she's only now considering how her confidence in her ability to handle her health problems might adversely affect her health status. Since she's so used to these problems and hates losing her composure in front of people, she often drives herself to the ER using one arm and patiently waits for someone to pop her shoulder back into place. She appears so calm and stoic that the triage staff often assume she isn't really in that much pain or that there isn't anything wrong with her, and she ends up waiting for a longer time as a result. Perhaps if she'd been "new" to chronic illness and wasn't so used to the cycle of injury, pain, and recovery, she would have manifested a more dramatic reaction, one that would have necessitated more immediate care, and ultimately, more immediate relief.

Like the physicians who listen to our symptoms and decide on courses of actions, most of the time, we're perfectly justified in our assumptions and disavowals—after all, we're the ones with the experience. Every now and then, though, it pays to stop assuming you have all the answers and run your symptoms by your doctors.

6.

THE WAITING GAME

Waiting is inevitable, but discern
when it is justified

W E'RE GOING TO ADMIT YOU, but you'll probably be in the ER for twenty to twenty-six hours before we can get you into a room." "Would you mind coming back to the lab tomorrow? We dropped a vial of your blood and need to run all the tests over again." "We won't be able to schedule a follow-up appointment to look at your results for three months. Do you want to be notified if there are any cancellations?" Sound familiar? If any other business operated with such poor customer service, it wouldn't last, but as patients, we put up with it because sometimes we have little choice. Waiting is yet another occupational hazard of living with illness. Rather than rail against the frustration, learn to distinguish which battles are worth fighting and which ones cause you more harm than benefit, and which delays are inevitable and which ones are unnecessary.

On visits to a certain doctor, I know I will have to wait at least a couple of hours for my scheduled appointment. In fact, I plan on it and always bring lots of work to keep me occupied. It's frustrating and inconvenient and usurps a lot of my free time, but I don't complain or nag the receptionist or gripe to the people around me about how long I've been waiting. Am I just preternaturally patient? Not a chance. But I do know this doctor well, and I know that if one of her patients requires an extended visit, a long conversation, or multiple interventions right there in the office, she will make time for that patient's needs. I have been that patient whose complicated symptoms required all that time, and I have been the patient she squeezed into an already booked schedule because I was too acute to wait. I remind myself of that when I start to get irritated—I've used up plenty of other patients' valuable time, so I can't complain when it's my turn to wait. If I were a new patient, chances are I would be one of the red-faced people making constant trips to the receptionist station to remind them of what time my appointment was supposed to be, but the benefit of experience means I don't expend that energy anymore.

If you have a condition that sometimes necessitates trips to the ER, then undoubtedly you've had a lengthy wait to be admitted to a room. A trip to the ER is practically synonymous with taxing one's patience. After all these years, I've learned to anticipate such waits, especially since my hospitals are large, urban teaching hospitals that serve huge numbers of people every day. They have only so many beds, and while I hate setting up camp in an ER bay or, during especially bad trips, on a gurney in a hallway somewhere, there's not much point in complaining—after all, the nurses and doctors want me to leave the ward as much as I do, because there is always a ready stream of patients waiting for my spot.

As the gatekeeper to the ER, the triage station is a powerful element of the evaluation-treatment cycle. (The only upside—and I say this with a heavy inference of irony—to arriving in the ER in a near-cyanotic state is that I am usually rushed back to a bay immediately. As a general rule, they try to avoid letting patients turn blue in the middle of a crowded waiting room.) If you have broken bones or other symptoms requiring attention and it is midnight on Saturday, you have little choice but to use the ER, knowing you have several hours of waiting ahead of you. And it makes sense, because the whole point of triaging patients is to weed out those who are in critical condition from those who may be uncomfortable but are not in danger—at least, that's how it's supposed to work. One of my more humorous triage experiences occurred when I was living in Dublin, Ireland, during my junior year in college and broke my ankle. The "triage" consisted of taking a number from a dispenser similar to the ones at deli counters and simply waiting for your number to be called. I hobbled over to a seat, where I wondered if the guy groaning next to me was having a heart attack or just had a stomachache. Since our numbers weren't weighted or prioritized, there was no way to tell.

As someone who has spent her fair share of time in the ER, Angela has a decidedly levelheaded approach to the entire process. "Some people say the squeaky wheel gets the grease, but I don't think complaining to the triage nurse about your wait—unless there's a change in your condition—while they have their hands full with gunshots and car accidents will shorten the wait, perhaps the opposite," she says.

However, her experiences also reveal a huge problem that is largely unique to chronically ill patients—the curse of being labeled a "regular," especially if what's causing your frequent trips is uncommon or misunderstood. For example, before Angela's second shoulder surgery in college, she had had an unusually large amount of dislocations, and, as such, she became known as a "frequent flier" to her local ER. Even if her shoulder injury was visible to the naked eye and the pain caused her to vomit and her blood pressure to sky-rocket, nurses would still sometimes roll their eyes to each other and say, "It's *her* again," and dismiss the severity of her problem. In triage-speak, this translates to being placed at the bottom of the interminable line of patients and exempli-fies the frustrating kind of treatment that shouldn't be toler-ated as status quo. Being overwhelmed by catastrophic injuries or a high volume of seriously ill patients is entirely understandable; being indifferent or altogether dismissive of a patient's condition and complaints is unacceptable.

"I've never come across a nurse who has heard of Ehlers-Danlos syndrome, but there's a difference between the ones who asked me what it is, and understood that it's the reason for my ridiculously frequent shoulder dislocations, and the ones who looked at me skeptically then scribbled down something phonetically close, not even bothering to spell it correctly. Medical professionals who fell into the latter category were the ones to treat me as if I was malingering or drug-seeking—despite the fact that I often refused narcotics and prescriptions for narcotics," Angela says.

This highlights a problem faced by patients across the disease spectrum: the ER isn't designed to cater to those with rare or complex diseases; specialists are. As patients, we can't expect ER staff to recognize our ailments immedi-ately, but we can, and *should*, expect them to take a few minutes to listen and process what we're saying.

Questions of supply and demand and triage and treat-ment aside, there are more annoying and little-mentioned aspects of waiting that shouldn't be ignored. Personally, I find dealing with the attitudes of other patients a lot more tiresome than the waiting itself—and like being in an over-crowded ER ward on a weekend night, there's not much I can do about it, save tempering my emotions. I once was in the ER at the same time as a drunken college student who swore and screamed repeatedly about the cut on his hand being ignored. He yelled assorted epitaphs and vulgarities at everyone from the triage nurse to the security guard, who threatened to remove him from the hospital. His behavior made a bad situation worse, not just for me but also for the poor pregnant girl next to me in obvious pain and the cry-ing family waiting to be allowed back to see their mother.

"That's just what all these sick, stressed people need: a loudmouthed punk," I muttered to my husband in between coughs and wheezes. Indignant as I was, there was nothing I could do except try to ignore him and continue waiting for my name to be called.

We wait for our turn to see the doctor, or for our blood to be drawn, or for our IVs to be inserted. We wait for lab results and appointment cancellations, and we wait for busy emergency room personnel to call our name. We wait because it is what we have to do to feel better; we hold our tongues where appropriate because it is what we have to do in order to not feel worse.

7.

SALIENT SUFFERING

*It isn't noble, it doesn't belong in the
world of platitudes, but suffering has
its place—and its merits*

W HEN I STUMBLED ACROSS THE FACT that the
word *patient* derives from the root "to suffer," I
was alternately amused and somewhat vindicated. As the
word's origin reveals, being a patient implies at least some
degree of suffering. As a general rule, I consider the word
suffering to be as emotionally and intellectually loaded as I
find the term *patient*. I fear it's too easy to lump together
platitudes about those who are sick—that we are somehow
stronger or better people for having endured pain or
extreme obstacles; that because we're sick, we're martyrs
and capable of serenely accepting challenges, setbacks, and
procedures without complaint.

Vicki, who is awaiting a double lung transplant, has
come to some pretty definitive realizations about what it
means to be a patient by this stage in her life. "I don't find

anything, *anything*, redemptive about being sick," she says. For years, people have told her how brave she is, how strong and resilient she must be to endure the many complications of her illness. They are likely referring to her ever-present cough, her intrusive feeding tube, or her very basic struggle to get enough air—all part of her daily life—when they make such comments. Some people assume that by virtue of these physical symptoms, Vicki is somehow naturally equipped to handle them. She disagrees with this all-too-common assumption, one that is as dangerous as it is flawed. She puts up with the disruptions and the bodily complaints because she *has* to, something perhaps healthy people don't always consider. If they were suddenly thrust into a similar situation, what else would they do but the things necessary for their health, and in cases like Vicki's, their survival?

Very often, illness doesn't allow the luxury of courage; pragmatism and practicality dictate the extent of our fearlessness. Throughout my childhood, I remember adults telling my mother what a "trooper" I was. They called me a fighter, but ultimately I didn't do anything particularly miraculous or noteworthy. When my ears gushed blood and infected pus and surgery was the only thing that stopped it, I submitted to the surgeries my parents scheduled without fanfare. I didn't view these surgeries as proof that I was courageous or tough; I was a little kid who wanted to feel better. As an adult, when my muscles feel weak and my brain starts to get foggy or I gasp for air because I can't stop coughing, I take the medications whose side effects I hate because that's all there is left to do. There is very little room for interpretation, inspiration, or intrepidness in these situations.

"I used to think that suffering makes you a better person, but it doesn't. It just makes you a better sufferer," Vicki says, placing a markedly candid spin on the nature of suffering. "At this point, I don't need anything else to enhance my character or prove I can handle a lot." Such a sentiment is inevitable, really. Chronic illness is never going to stop presenting challenges and our bodies are never going to stop surprising us with new manifestations of illness, so to some degree, we're all going to face the "enough is enough" moment.

So what does it mean to be a "better sufferer"? That you cry less when things are painful, that you get less angry when you experience another loss? That choices, from small things like when to call a doctor to life-altering decisions like putting yourself on a transplant list, are somehow made easier once you've reached a certain threshold? Does it mean that things physically hurt less or that invasive procedures are somehow less invasive if you've been through it before? Hardly.

Suffering doesn't make you a better person, in the sense that a person with these challenges is somehow more noble or "good" in a moral way. But I think there's another dimension to this notion of being a better sufferer, one stripped of greeting-card-inspired platitudes and skewed interpretations of what it means to live with illness. The more you suffer, the more you are able to recognize suffering in others. The fact that our experiences make us privy to this knowledge is a privilege I think gets lost in the "suffering saint" attributes of illness, but what we do with that knowledge is what really counts. We're not better people because we can empathize with someone's struggle with infertility or migraines or because we can nod our heads in understanding when someone is frustrated about a diagnosis or a side effect. However, if we are able to channel accumulated patient experiences in a way that somehow makes a positive impact on someone else in a similar situation, then there is something redemptive about our suffering.

8.

THE INSTITUTION INVADES THE LIVING ROOM

*The daily intrusion of illness in our
private lives is a necessary—and
worthwhile—evil*

MOST CHRONIC ILLNESSES HAVE their own unique method of intruding on our personal lives. It's one thing to deal with the medical establishment when you're at the doctor's office or in the hospital, but it's another thing to have that establishment follow you home. From visiting nurses to the people who come to our houses to demonstrate how insulin pumps work to the actual devices like pumps and blood pressure cuffs that clutter up our living space, there are always reminders of illness.

So what do you do when the trappings of illness invade your personal space?

I'll admit that when I first found out in 2003 that I needed a physical therapist to perform chest physiotherapy (chest PT) on me every single day for the rest of my life, I was less than ecstatic. I didn't mind the numerous medications I needed to take daily. I was used to my nebulizer and assorted inhalers and breathing paraphernalia. But chest PT was a whole different beast, and I was much less tractable. What really bothered me was that now there was no clear demarcation between illness as an institution and illness as something private and personal. I couldn't go home, close my door, and leave that other sterile, clinical world of doctors and practitioners behind me anymore, not when a physical therapist showed up at my house every day, sometimes twice a day.

A typical chest PT session lasts about half an hour and consists of a therapist cupping his or her hands and "clapping" the lobes of the lungs in eleven exact positions—shoulders, clavicle, upper back, lower back, sides, the spot where the breast bone meets the underarm, the ribs, and the chest itself. Some positions are performed while sitting in a chair, others while sprawled in various poses on a couch or bed. Each spot receives about two minutes of clapping followed by vibrations, which are when the hands compress down quickly side to side, squeezing air in and out of the mucus in the lobes. The irony of chest PT is that the worse you feel after it—the more hacking your cough and more choking your phlegm—the better it is working.

As a chest PT virgin, I had no idea what to expect during my first session. It was August 2003, just weeks after I'd been discharged from the ICU and walked away from my old hospital and my old doctors forever. I was attending a good-bye party for a friend at a bar later that night and was already dressed for the evening when Steve, my therapist, arrived. I wore a long, flared denim skirt, a blue shirt with a V-neck and a white collar, and tottering butterscotch leather heels that added about five inches to my five-foot-one stature. It was my favorite summer outfit, and since I'd spent much of the summer in the hospital, I was determined to maximize it.

I couldn't have been more ill-prepared for the next half hour.

Chest PT *hurt*. As in gritting-my-teeth, holding-my-breath, I-will-not-complain-even-if-it-kills-me-which-it-just-might hurt. Huge welts and deep bruises sprang up almost immediately after Steve got to work on my sides and my ribs, especially where the skin is most sensitive, right where the armpit meets the breast tissue.

My blue shirt kept riding up when I was facedown on the couch, and when I turned to lie on my side, my skirt got all twisted and tangled and I knew Steve could see my underwear. Worst of all, no one had told me that someone would be whacking away basically right where my breasts were (I should have assumed, but still), particularly from the side, and I could feel them bouncing up and down with each rhythmic clap. I was mortified and swore I'd wear a sports bra every session from that point forward. *Please God, let him be gay. This is too awkward. Please let him be gay.* I pleaded over and over in my head, counting the seconds till I could right myself again, cheeks flushed.

I never had such modesty in clinical settings, but there was something so uncomfortably intimate about a total stranger seeing me in such a vulnerable position in my own home. I had always been the one in control of my health in my own place, and now it was clear I needed outside help to do the job. It took me a long time to chip away at my resentment toward chest PT—with up to two sessions a day, seven days a week, fifty-two weeks a year, the constant demand on my time felt like an anchor holding me back, not something that would move me forward. I had considered my home a respite, and now more than ever, illness was an unavoidable part of my daily life.

But I had to admit it helped. That was the great incentive for integrating chest PT, or any other time-consuming but productive treatment therapy we might need. Within a few weeks of starting chest PT, I could tell I was moving more air. After three weeks to a month, when the skin had toughened up a bit and callused and the new bruises had finally stopped swelling, it didn't hurt as much, although it still was inconvenient and unpleasant. During that first winter with chest PT, my hospitalizations decreased from seven or eight to four or five. How could I argue with something that ultimately allowed me to feel better? Wasn't it worth the sacrifice in time and energy day to day if it meant losing less time to "sick" days and hospitalizations? Gradually, the rational patient in me returned, and just as I knew all the pills, inhalers, and sprays I took every day were worth whatever inconvenience because they helped me manage my conditions, I knew chest PT was no different.

I also began to realize that I could keep viewing Steve's presence as intrusion, or I could stop being stubborn and start seeing him as a connection to the outside world that I sometimes had to leave when I wasn't feeling well. We all know how isolating prolonged spells at home recuperating can be. Whether he was aware of it or not, beyond giving necessary therapy, Steve had become an integral part of my daily life. On my "bad" days, when I was housebound and isolated, he provided a fresh face to break up the long, wheezy hours, a link to the flurry of the outside world besides the constant whir and hum of my laptop. It is my vulnerability—something even some of my closest friends don't have access to but on the rarest of occasions—that makes the bond between him and me such a unique one.

There are countless ways illness breaks into the peaceful escape we'd like to believe we have at home. But perhaps our homes are the very best places to confront our illness—we're on our own turf and we know that every treatment, medication, or clinician we let inside our doors is there because we have made that choice. Such treatments and visual signs of illness aren't so much outside forces destroying our sanctuaries as they are tools that enable us to feel well enough to leave our private world of illness when we see fit.

9.

BILINGUAL PATIENTS

*Fluency in hospital-speak is the best
means of survival*

HOME MIGHT BE THE SANCTUARY temporarily inter-
rupted by illness, but hospitals are the epicenter of
the sick existence. If anything spells victory over daunting
forces, it's the ability to evince humor in an otherwise difficult situation like a prolonged hospitalization. Hospitals
are obviously places where serious and often scary health
events occur—there's a reason why so many people hate going to them. But for those of us who have no choice but to
frequent them, there is a way to survive hospitals with our
sanity and sense of humor intact. Instead of questioning the
counterintuitive logic of hospitals, embrace it. You need to
become fluent in hospital-speak, a code of phrases and alternative meanings for otherwise ordinary terms. It really is
comparable to speaking a foreign language—until you have
the idioms and customary phrases of a hospital down, you
will never truly acclimate.

Washing Up

In my mind, the pristine phrase "washing up" conjures up wholesome images of *Little House on the Prairie* with Michael Landon and Melissa Gilbert beaming at each other as they rinse their hands off in the metal pail before sitting down to steaming bowls of potatoes and Ma's cured ham. All those warm, fuzzy feelings dissipate when you enter the hospital's take on "washing up." Typically, you are given a number of scratchy towels in various sizes, a kidney-shaped bin of lukewarm water that quickly turns tepid, a miniature bar of soap, and a toothbrush. Some people opt for a nurse to assist them with washing up, and while there is less chance of tangled wires or tubing in that scenario than when you try it on your own, it still doesn't do much for the hair situation.

My mother insists on wearing full makeup when she's an inpatient, as if reapplying fuschia lipstick and blue eye shadow throughout the day somehow makes her fresher or cleaner. I can understand her logic—the old "you'll feel better if you look better" line of thought—and until she tried to apply bright pink rouge to my face when I was the patient, I found this habit of hers charming. The bottom line? Use the bar of soap when and where you can, don't expect anything but matted, greasy hair, and remember that a roll of deodorant can accomplish almost as much as the ill-conceived washing up.

The Commode

While current usage dictates that "toilet" and "commode" are practically interchangeable, in the hospital you'd never mistake using the toilet (the porcelain bowl that resides in its own little room) for using the commode (a rickety little chamber pot on wheels). The word *commode* sounds so classy, so foreign and sophisticated, but in reality, slapping a self-compressing seat over a plastic tray and balancing it atop a walker isn't exactly refined. Using a commode in the middle of the hospital room is a lot like fat-free cheese slices: all wrong and too unnatural. An even more undignified function of the hospital commode occurs when visitors use your closed commode for a seat before you can stop them. Laugh as you may, but I've seen it happen. Remember, nurses are busy and can't always empty things right away. A closed commode does not mean it is a *clean* commode, so be on guard.

Excavation and the Butterfly Needle

When an exasperated lab tech inserts a needle for a second time and still no blood enters the blood test tube, it can only mean one thing: *excavation*. No, we aren't on some far-flung *National Geographic* expedition in Nepal; we're talking about someone digging around inside your arm with a needle, pushing, prodding, and jabbing to try to locate a vein that hasn't rolled away or collapsed. The only things phlebotomists can use for such veins are butterfly needles, which are so small they can't possibly overwhelm an exhausted little vein. My father, who has terrible veins and the unfortunate propensity as a diabetic heart patient to need a lot of blood drawn, is a butterfly-only kind of guy. When a blood technician enters his room, my father will firmly but politely say, "Only use the butterfly needle, please." Sometimes, technicians will shrug him off with gallant phrases like "Oh, you only say that because you've never had blood drawn by me before. You'll see, we don't need a butterfly." After a few rounds of this back-and-forth, my father's response is inevitably: "Do. Not. Stick. Me. With. Anything. But. A. Butterfly." His smile turns into a pursed-lip stare, and suddenly there are no more quipping protests from anyone else in the room. The man knows his needles.

Environmental Control

Whenever I hear the phrase "environmental control," I think of people in white haz-mat suits scurrying around and cordoning off quarantine areas, much like the frenzied scenes in the movie *Outbreak*. The real-life notion of environmental control is more oxymoronic than Hollywood's version. When you gather the most contagious and infectious people in one place and inevitably expose them to each other, there's no way antibacterial hand lotion in each room and public health signs urging everyone to cover their mouth when they cough can contain the germs. You'd like to believe all the floor mopping and hand washing means hospitals are disinfected, but humans aren't even the only threats in the battle for germ security: I've had stays where my roommates were cheeky, aggressive city mice. Nothing says "sterile environment" like mice dancing around your IV pole. I was told the environmental control office was aware of the rodent situation, but the mice sure didn't look worried. I have a good friend with several serious illnesses who absolutely refuses to go to the hospital in her town. She'd rather hole herself up in the cocoon of her living room and manage her life-threatening symptoms from there. "They'd kill me in the hospital. Between not knowing how to handle my conditions and all the germs, I'd never come out of there

alive," she said once with a laugh that, like most laughs relating to hospitals, was part genuine and part acquiescent.

The ICU

When you're one of the healthier patients in the ICU—an
irony in itself, to be sure—the term more accurately means
"intensive confinement unit," something akin to a prison
but with lots of monitors and tubes as an added bonus.
There may be a jack in the wall, but there is no phone or
phone cord for computer hookup, and cell phones are
banned. Visitors are allowed, but they only trickle in one
or two at a time and are monitored frequently by the nursing staff to ensure there aren't too many all at once. The
lights are usually switched off and curtains drawn no matter what time it is, so reading, should you feel up to it, is
not a possibility. There is a TV remote next to the call but-
ton, but only a few channels come in and someone is always turning the volume down so low you can't hear it.
Since no real connection with the outside world is possible
in the intensive confinement unit, I've learned to pack an
extra phone cord so that when no one is looking, I can
hook up my laptop to the Internet via the dial-up method.
Like a prisoner hiding contraband razor blades, I cover the
stealth computer with my blanket and rest my IV-laden
arm over the bulge whenever nurses enter the room and
bide my time until I can be released into the general population once more.

"The Team"

You're imagining football players in spiffy uniforms break-ing out of a huddle when you see the word *team*, aren't you? Not in hospital-speak. In a teaching hospital, you aren't a member of your medical team so much as you are the human football. Med students, interns, and residents use your body to gain knowledge, and while you obviously benefit from this process, you also give up something huge along the way: modesty. "Do you mind if all the team members palpate your spleen? It would be helpful for them to feel it," and "Do you mind pulling down your johnny so the team can really hear your breath sounds from different positions?" are common team requests. By the end of a hospitalization, I feel like half the world has seen me naked or otherwise compromised. When I was in college, I would run into members of my team in line at the campus coffee shop adjacent to the hospital, which was decidedly awkward. We'd exchange sheepish nods of recognition, and I'd grab my nonfat mocha latte and run. Whenever you're playing with the team, it's best to re-peat the mantra "They have seen it all before" and try to believe it—once you realize the spectrum of disgusting things the team has witnessed, you'll laugh at the notion that your nakedness was anything special.

Familiarity

In most contexts, familiarity is a good thing: the guy in the coffee shop who knows your usual order, the neighbor who smiles as you walk your dog, the hostess who seats you at your favorite table. In hospital-speak, familiarity signifies the top echelon of proficiency, but it is probably the most

bittersweet term because it implies complete and total surrender to the alternative universe of the hospital. There are
numerous telltale signs that true familiarity has been attained: You go for an outpatient checkup and everyone from
the security guards to the radiologist on a smoke break rec-
ognizes you, or you're wheeled onto a floor and the nurses
smile and tell you your favorite room has an open bed.
There are also smaller, more personal signs you have
reached familiarity. You catch a whiff of rubbing alcohol
outside the door and, like me, by the time the lab tech has
entered, you have shoved forward your "best" vein and have
already begun pumping your tightly clenched fist to facili-
tate the blood draw, or you spot a stethoscope on a neck and
automatically untie your johnny in the back and lean forward. At this point, you have passed the ultimate proficiency
exam—you're so fluent in the language and terminology
that you don't even need to think about it anymore and react
purely on instinct.

10.

INSTITUTIONAL AUTHORITY

*No one's word is sacrosanct; don't be
afraid to speak up in the hospital*

IT'S ONE THING TO EXERT YOUR VOICE when you're at
a doctor's appointment, to reassert symptoms a physician
may have skipped over or to second-guess an opinion or con-
clusion. In these types of situations, you're typically dealing
with one other person, your doctor, and both of you usually
have working knowledge of your health status. But what
about when you're in the hospital, when you're acutely ill
and hordes of different people wearing scrubs of different
colors and white coats of different lengths come in and out of
your room? It's much more difficult to speak up then. Yet for
these very reasons, the hospital is the one place where it is
most imperative never to take anyone's authority for granted.

I've had enough blunders in my career as a patient to
know that many things that can go awry in a hospital. Some
of my most notable mishaps? When I was thirteen, I woke up
during a surgery. In my post-anesthesia haze I assumed the

incident was a dream, that I had imagined feeling like I was suffocating and trying to rip out the tube that was down my throat. But the sheepish apologies of my attending physician and the anesthesiologist confirmed it had actually happened. I've been left upside down and forgotten about during a barium swallow test, the oxygen I needed on the other side of the room where it was rendered fairly useless. I've even been sent for another patient's brain CT scan, despite my repeated (and emphatic) insistence that my head was fine and my infection-filled lungs were the problem. If I hadn't felt so weak, I'd have physically removed myself from the room and from the radiologist who kept telling me that I was wrong and that my orders called for a brain scan. Instead, I complained about the incident once I was oxygenated and fully indignant. It took a lot of work for my attending physician at the time to get the phrase "patient has altered mental status" out of my medical record, since I was not in fact the patient with the brain tumor and the altered mental status.

These are the more outrageous but completely factual events that have happened to me as a hospital patient, the "war stories" that usually entertain as well as slightly horrify interested parties. My point isn't to induce fear so much as to underscore the need to be vigilant in a setting where there are so many people and moving parts involved in your care. The most common types of mistakes I see are miscommunications between the floor nurses and doctors and the physical therapy team, which means I don't get the chest PT or nebulizer treatment I need. I don't like having to repeat my requests over and over, but I know what the doctor's orders are and what I am supposed to have, and it's my duty to make sure what is written for me actually happens for me. Likewise, I know exactly which drugs I cannot tolerate and have had to be quite vocal when they somehow wind up getting prescribed for me anyway. I'm not about to take a pill I know will make me vomit relentlessly just because someone tells me I'm supposed to take it, especially when there are obvious alternatives.

Another type of problem stems from the fact that many adult hospitals are not used to treating diseases that, until quite recently, most people didn't survive with into adulthood. It's one of the most significant trends I see emerging in medicine: better technology means chronically ill kids grow up and enter an adult system unprepared for them. Brian's experience with this is especially pertinent for the hundreds of thousands of patients with diseases that, like his cystic fibrosis, have better treatments and longer life expectancies than ever before. As a member of one of the first waves of CF "kids" to enter an adult cystic fibrosis program, Brian has witnessed the steep learning curve for health care professionals firsthand. During one hospital stay, he was almost given a dose of a particularly toxic medicine that was much too high—so high it would have put him at risk for liver failure. He intervened before it was too late, but that entire hospitalization was unusually miserable and protracted for him.

"I hate that, when you have to stop someone. You have to pay so much attention to what they're doing," Brian says. And it isn't always easy to be vigilant when you're especially weak or fatigued. It was never something he had to worry about when he was a pediatric patient in a CF ward, surrounded by patients just like him and nurses well acquainted with the standard treatment for CF patients and their complications. In the two years he's been in an adult program, he says he's definitely seen improvement in medical staff understanding and anticipating his needs, but he remains highly alert for any breaches in protocol in terms of the treatment regimen he knows so well.

We know the nuances of our bodies and our conditions more intimately than anyone else—and the more unfamiliar our conditions, the more important that point becomes. As Angela points out, "Having a rare disorder like EDS, which is only given brief mention in most medical textbooks, makes matters even worse, since many physicians are not at all familiar with the syndrome and its complications, and either don't have the time or won't take the time to look it up before addressing my complaint." As evidence of this, she relates the story of one ER physician who ordered a set of X-rays to confirm her shoulder was back in its socket. She feared one of the positions required for a certain view would likely dislocate the joint, given the ligament laxity and tears she had. In response, she was told she was being paranoid. Of course, she was right—taking the X-ray from that angle caused the shoulder to pop right back out again.

"I should have trusted my knowledge of my faulty connective tissue and my experience with that shoulder over the opinion of the physician, who was either unfamiliar with characteristics of EDS or was treating me without taking it into account. After that experience, I always refused to have an X-ray taken in that position, sometimes to the consternation of the ordering physician," she says.

What all these stories share is an underlying premise that it is far too easy for the patient voice to get lost in the complicated structure of hospitals. It can be difficult to question the authority of the highly trained medical professionals we encounter in hospitals, but there are times when we need to do just that. After all, the larger and more complex the system, the more likely it is that confusion can take root.

11.

HUMANIZING HOSPITALS

*There are ways to cater to the whole
patient in the hospital*

I'VE JOKED THAT THERE should be some sort of a
hospital frequent-flier program to reward valued
patients—the more visits, the more perks you acquire.
While there is no gold card membership or accrued points
redeemable for gifts, if you spend enough time on the same
ward, you eventually become a person, not simply a patient,
and there are benefits to this. From fluffier pillows to extra
diet ginger ale to lenient visiting hours, the staff will often
look the other way when it is obvious that slight infractions
actually do more to heal you than enforcing rules would—
it's up to you to recognize that there is room for humanity
in the hospital setting.

There is no lonelier time on earth than three A.M. in a
hospital ward. Most other patients have drifted off into listless sleep, the nurses' station is eerily quiet, and the predawn
blood draws—is it possible to look forward to them for the

sheer distraction?—have not yet begun. All that remains is muted darkness and the knowledge that, however comfortable the staff has tried to make you, you are not at home. If ever there are times I feel removed from the healthy world, these nights are the epitome of that isolation.

Of all the long, sleepless hospital nights I've had, one in particular stands out. It was spring of my sophomore year in college, and I was wide awake from a combination of pain and stimulants. I was restless, anxious, and exhausted. The late-night talk shows were over and the early-morning news shows had not started; only infomercials for Windsor Pilates and 1-800-Hot Young Blondes were on at that hour. In disgust, I muted the television so that only its light kept me company. My door was slightly ajar, and a thin crack of light came in from the hallway. I caught traces of passing conversations, heard an idle resident flip through a chart and snap it back in its binder, and heard a nurse discuss her daughter's upcoming wedding. Out my window I had a clear view of my campus apartment complex across the street; even most of the college kids had their lights out by now. I strained to see if there was any sign of life in my five-person unit on the ground floor, but all looked quiet and still.

During the day I thrived on the act of being a good patient, of smiling at the appropriate times for the appropriate people and reassuring everyone that I was okay. Keeping up this elaborate front gave me something to do. In the morning, the show was for doctors and students on rounds; if I performed well enough, maybe they would agree to send me home. In the afternoon and evening, the show was geared toward friends and roommates who visited. But in those lost hours between rounds and visitors, there was no one left to act for, and I was left alone with my own thoughts and fears.

I watched the second hand tick off the minutes: 3:15 . . . 3:30. Only an hour and half till the early-morning news would come on and I could put on the volume. Only two hours till the morning blood draw. Only four hours till rounds, and maybe I could leave. *Who was I kidding?* Still, I could make it four hours longer. These thoughts raced in and out of my head, jumbled with worries about missing too much school before finals, whether I remembered to drop off the disk with my feature article at the newspaper office, how much longer this particular IV would remain in my arm before it got infected.

I heard a faint tap at the door and mumbled, "Come in." I assumed it was time for the nurse to check my vitals, so I didn't even look up.

"Hey, sweetie. You're awake. How are you?" In the doorway stood my close friend Jason. It was a warm, muggy night and he was wearing a T-shirt I loved, bright orange with a thin blue and white strip across the chest. It was a shirt so loud that on most people it would seem ostentatious; on Jason, it just worked. I loved that he could pull off such a shirt, mainly because I never could—one of the many differences between the two of us. He wore his baggy carpenter jeans and had a textbook and a ballpoint pen in his right hand. His brown eyes looked at me inquisitively.

"Hey! What are you doing here? It's so late! How did you get in?" I straightened up in my bed and readjusted my johnny, which had shifted down below my left shoulder. I wiped my eyes, trying to hide any traces of tears.

"I knew you'd be awake. And alone. And I'd rather be with you than thinking of you here all night with no one. I was up writing this paper anyway, so I figured, why not?"

"And they didn't hassle you at security? Or the nurses' station?"

"A little, but I wouldn't take no for an answer. And here I am." He pulled the pink leather chair up to my bedside and sat down, grasping my hand and stroking it lightly.

"So tell me, dear, how are you? How's your breathing?" he asked. It is our running joke that I keep forgetting how to breathe. *In, out, in, out*, he reminds me.

"I'm okay. A lot better now that you're here. I can't even believe it. You have so much work to do, really you don't need to be here," I said, wanting him to leave so I wouldn't feel so guilty and thrilled he was there at the same time.

"I don't *need* to do anything. I want to be here."

With most people, I still might have thought they were saying this to placate me. But with Jason, I knew it was the truth, and I relaxed.

For the first time in six nights, I drifted off to sleep for a little while, Jason's hand still resting on top of mine. I woke up around 4:45 when I heard soft footsteps; my night nurse stood in the doorway and smiled. Jason was fast asleep, his other hand still clutching his textbook and pen. I watched his chest rise and fall.

In, out, in, out. It looked so easy.

The nurses at my university's medical center had always been somewhat lenient with me and my entourage of visitors—they looked the other way when large groups of people would file in as long as we were quiet. They scrounged up binders full of takeout menus so hungry friends could have food delivered. They helped me arrange the towering stack of textbooks and binders my roommates brought me so that they were within my reach yet not in the way of the tubes and monitors. They knew I got clammy and sweaty from the steroids and they always made sure I had fresh, dry sheets. I firmly believe that the nurses, not the doctors or anyone else, are the ones who truly define a patient's stay—they are the ones who spend the most time with us and attend to our needs when we can't.

This particular night, Jason's friendship was obviously the greatest gift, the link I so desperately needed to the outside world. I don't like the fact that I am a "frequent flier," but if I am going to spend so much time in hospitals, I am glad that there are nurses who take the time to learn my preferences and idiosyncrasies—and visitors who are willing to forgo a night's sleep in their own bed to sit by my side.

12.

HOSPITAL HUB

Hospitalizations may be inevitable
but surrendering your personality
doesn't have to be

W HEN I AM IN THE EMERGENCY ROOM, as soon as
the flurry of immediate help subsides, which basically means as soon as I am capable of breathing enough to
speak, my first question is always the same: "When can I go
home?" I cajole, negotiate, and wheedle my way out of being admitted whenever possible, and the usual response to
my repeated inquiries is something along the lines of, "You
just got here and already you're talking about when you can
go home?"

Of course I am. No matter the condition that brings you
to the hospital, there is nothing more disrupting than an extended stay, and like many of you, I've spent too many
weeks of my life as an inpatient to want to remain there for
one minute longer than absolutely necessary. So much of
the daily maintenance, the medications and appointments,

and the general heightened level of attention we pay to our health is often to avoid this very situation, when our conditions flare beyond our ability to manage them on our own. For so many different illnesses, from Crohn's disease and colitis to endocrine or metabolic disorders, hospitalizations are inevitable realities of chronic life.

Clearly the hospital is the ultimate physical embodiment of medicine as an institution. We might not be able to avoid the institution, but there are ways to withstand its rigors without total surrender to it. After all these years, I've concocted my own particular breed of defiance, my way of remaining in control when I am an inpatient and virtually everything—how much oxygen I have, where I go to the bathroom, what fluids I intake—is out of my hands. Two decades' worth of time spent in hospitals and much discussion with other patients have shown me that each person's response is as idiosyncratic as his or her particular manifestation of illness. But how we respond to hospitalizations is much less important than the basic presupposition that we *do* respond.

I have my own version of the "pregnant lady suitcase," a backpack whose contents can be pulled together within five minutes. As soon as I start feeling that the-hospital-just-may-be-in-my-future pit in my stomach, I make sure the essential items are near: laptop, power cord, Ethernet cable and extra phone cord, glasses and glasses case, deodorant, face wash, underwear and socks, hairbrush, cell phone and charger, magazines. Oh, and my medicines, of course, because the hospital pharmacy doesn't always have what I take and it is more efficient and less expensive to just bring my own pills and inhalers than to have the nursing staff try to hunt them down and dole them out several times a day. As evidenced by what I consider necessities, my agenda in the hospital is to ignore the fact that I can't breathe and have a pesky IV line in my arm as much as possible and to create a home office environment. Whether it's the stimulants pumped into me to stabilize my airways, the constant cough that keeps me awake, or my well-established tendency toward compulsion, I choose to view extended hospitalizations as an opportunity to get work done. Once my visitors leave, I'm all work, all the time. Of course I don't feel well and of course it's hard to concentrate when I'm in pain, but except for the most serious infections and flares when I'm just too weak, I figure I'd rather be miserable and productive than just miserable. Knowing I am away from work or classes is much less stressful if I can keep up on my own, a remnant from a childhood spent missing huge amounts of school.

Evidence of my somewhat zealous crusade? With the help of the Internet, I've gotten an apartment, a job, and recruited several writers for a magazine I edited—all from my hospital bed. I've also written papers, studied for finals, taken conference calls for my college newspaper (oxygen mask and all), and planned elaborate holiday soirees, fund-raisers, and birthday parties as an inpatient. It is no coincidence that my intensity has increased the older I've gotten—from maintaining internships in college to working at my first "real" job to attending graduate school, the amount of time I spent in hospitals increased during the precise time in my life when I needed to focus on building a career.

I'm the kind of girl who has to-do lists for her to-do lists, who always hated group projects because I knew I could do a better job on my own, who wakes up in the middle of the night, suddenly remembering an edit I'd forgotten to make in a document. I've always chalked a lot of this perfectionist/control stuff up to the fact that I have always been so sick: I can't control so much about my life, so what I can control, I try to do in full force. I take the large issues, the life-threatening ones, in stride, so it's sometimes the smaller stuff that frustrates me. It makes sense, and it's certainly a convenient rationalization on days when I wish I could just escape myself a little bit.

More recently, I've started wondering about how much of my personality is defined by illness—or more accurately, a reaction to the presence of illness—and how much is just my personality. Would I be this way if I were healthy? Since I've never been healthy, I just don't know. I know that in various ways I am a lot like other patients I've met and a lot like my parents, but since illness is our common denominator, it's hard to tell. Even still, when I am hospitalized, I sleep with my laptop either nestled in my covers or anchored to the tray table, and I make covert cell phone calls once I'm sure there are no nurses around. Do I sound completely crazy? Perhaps, but the more my health pulls me away from what I want to do, the more ways I find to compensate for that. This approach might not appeal to everyone—certainly I know many people who prefer to watch TV or read books and magazines purely for entertainment, and that works just as well for them.

The spectrum of chronic illness is enormous, and obviously some diseases necessitate a lot more time in hospitals than others. For Vicki, being away from her home and the people she loves is distressing, and the rupture of the normalcy of her everyday life is draining. In response, she does whatever she can to make her room and her living conditions as close to her home as possible. She always brings her medications with her too, which not only saves a lot of time, money, and hassle but can even mean the difference between feeling better or getting worse; once the hospital pharmacy was out of the pancreatic enzyme CF patients like Vicki need to absorb nutrients and she couldn't eat.

Vicki also brings her own food and drinks and stores them in her own little fridge. This is partly emotional—her favorite foods and drinks are certainly more appealing than standard hospital cuisine—but is also pragmatic. The institution of medicine is inherently biased against the patient in the sense that in our most vulnerable state, we need the nurses, doctors, transport members, and lab techs a lot more than they need us. A self-proclaimed control freak, Vicki views as a necessary victory any little step that means she's not relying on other people to do things for her. Even something as small as the act of drinking her own juice when she wants it, rather than buzzing for a nurse to bring her some juice when the nurse has a chance, makes a difference to her.

While Vicki always makes sure she is polite and appreciative of her medical team in the hospital, she also establishes clear boundaries and is unwilling to sacrifice her sense of privacy and comfort for the academic goals of teaching hospitals. Anyone who has spent time in a teaching hospital knows how tiresome the team approach can be—how many times can you give your medical history in one day before you start to get a little irritated? Clearly we need teaching hospitals, and medicine is a science and a practice that depends on this hands-on type of learning. But what isn't as obvious to many patients—in fact, it's something I didn't even realize until Vicki told me—is that you don't always have to be a cog in the teaching hospital machine. For patients like Vicki who have no choice but to be hospitalized frequently, it makes a lot of sense to exercise this right. She no longer allows interns and residents to work with her when she's admitted.

"I'm not here to educate them; I'm here to get well," she says, emphasizing that her physical and emotional needs as a patient are more important than, say, a fourth-year medical student's desire to learn more about cystic fibrosis. In a way, this all ties in with her mini-fridge and her food and drinks—in the hospital, it's all about picking which things are most important to you as a person, not just as a patient, and doing whatever it takes to ensure these things are still within your grasp.

13.

THE WAITING ROOM AS THE GREAT EQUALIZER

Sometimes you learn the most about
illness when you're not the patient

A T FIRST, MY MOTHER and I were the only ones in the waiting room. Armed with magazines, books, and gluten-free energy bars in case our wait lasted several hours, we settled ourselves into the row of chairs in the far right corner of the room, the ones that faced the window. It was a brashly sunny day; I could practically see the sticky, suffocating August heat rising from the city street below. The banter of *Good Morning America* reached us from the television on the other side of the room, but aside from that, the only sound for a long time was the sloshing of ice cubes against plastic each time I picked up my iced coffee, took a sip, and placed it back down on the coffee table. We held our assorted magazines without reading them and watched the TV without listening. Only a few feet away, on the other side of the two automatic doors marked CARDIAC

CATHETERIZATION LAB, a tiny probe illuminated by iodine-based dye snaked its way from my father's femur up to his heart, searching out his blocked arteries, unfolding his fate.

As the daughter of two chronically ill parents, I thought I'd nailed the art of being a good visitor, although I most often played the role of patient. Whenever one of my parents was hospitalized, we reversed our positions and it was my turn to sit at the bedside, procure magazines and books, and ferry illicit cups of Dunkin Donuts coffee into my mother's or father's hospital room. It was during these times that I also appreciated my brothers' role in our nuclear family: whether it was my lungs, my father's heart or muscle diseases, or my mother's serious joint diseases, Michael and Marc have always been the ones who do the visiting, who juggle their own schedules and the needs of their own families to be there for us.

I'd always assumed that being a patient made me a more informed, knowledgeable visitor. What I didn't realize was how much being a visitor could teach me about being a patient. My father's catheterization was a delicate process made even more enervating because of his existing health conditions. I think I'd assumed that waiting for a loved one's procedure to be finished would be that much more terrifying for me if I didn't understand what was going on. I was wrong. I was overwhelmed by the enormity of what I *did* know and understand, the complex chain of consequences and scenarios we could not escape.

So my mother and I waited anxiously. By the time *The View* came on, more seats in the waiting room had filled up. Pretending to read the *New Yorker*, I focused my otherwise listless attention on the others in the room. To our right were a mother and daughter. I guessed the woman to be in her late forties and the girl to be in her late teens; I found out later that indeed the daughter would be starting her freshman year in college in a few weeks' time. They were loud, though not in an unpleasant way, and, within minutes of sitting down, they'd tired of talking to each other and inserted themselves into the wall of silence the rest of us had maintained.

Well before the mother said it was the first time her husband had experienced any health problems, I knew they'd never seen illness in their nuclear family. Everything seemed too new to them. They settled into the wooden chairs with expectant looks on their faces, not sure what to do or what would entertain them. They hadn't chosen the seats that faced the TV, nor had they brought reading material, knitting, crossword puzzles, or any of the usual paraphernalia people carry around with them in hospitals like protective shields. Instead, they chattered nervously when my mother and I engaged them in conversation, their statements ending with question marks that didn't belong, as if they were hoping we could validate or confirm what they'd been told as fact really was true: "It's a simple procedure, really?" and "Depending on what they find, if there isn't a big blockage, he could be released today, home for dinner?"

They explained to my mother—who hadn't asked, but listened with genuine empathy and patience—exactly what a catheterization was. *Don't they realize we know all of this? That we're all waiting for the same news?* I was incredulous, but not entirely irritated. I smiled, nodded, and "mmm hmmmed" where appropriate, leaving the bulk of the niceties to my mother. I felt a little protective of their wide-eyed innocence, enhanced by my belief that their loved one's cath would be uneventful and he would require no further intervention besides medication. Thankfully, that was one thing I was right about that day.

The elderly woman to our left had been equally swept

up in our conversation. Though she hadn't yet gotten a chance to discuss her own situation, I could tell she was a veteran. Her tote bag was open, revealing issues of *Reader's Digest*, a bottle of water, and an apple. I detected what I thought was a small grimace of pain when she shifted in her seat. Like me, she had a sweater on her lap; after a half hour or so in the blasting chill of the air-conditioned room, she draped it over her shoulders. The most telling sign, though, was her demeanor with the chatty pair. Just as my mother had been doing since the start, this woman nodded and re-assured the two in the right places and made polite small talk about where they came from, the weather, how nice the doctors and nurses in this hospital were. Whatever worry or stress she felt, she did not reveal. I wondered if she too felt somewhat protective of these two strangers who had stum-bled into our world.

The mother and the daughter were the first ones to leave the waiting room that morning, flush with the good news the doctors gave them. Once they were gone, my mother and the elderly woman became engrossed in their own conversation; their husbands' complicated medical histories and their own similar joint and rheumatologic problems serving as com-mon threads. Gradually, I put down my magazine altogether and joined in. The tenor of the conversation was different—it was more matter-of-fact, more direct; we did not worry about protecting each other from the fear we felt. At the same time, it was still a conversation rooted in the common mix of worry, hope, and distraction the mother and daughter had felt.

While we waited for my father, I thought a lot about all the different people in the room. For years I'd been so con-ditioned to view the world in extremes: either you were sick or you weren't, either you understood the alternate world of the hospital or you didn't. Such broad generalizations came from the perspective of a patient, someone so used to surgeries and risk-benefit analyses that I fooled myself into believing that being a seasoned patient somehow guaranteed that being a visitor would be easier. That long morning in the waiting room served as an equalizer for me, closing the gap I'd so earnestly believed existed between the healthy and the sick. All the experience and knowledge in the world doesn't count for much when we're the ones in the waiting room—no matter our backgrounds and experiences, we're all just people whose hope hinges on what's happening on the other side of the double-swinging doors.

14.
COMMUNITY HEALTH

*Recognize the value of the shared
patient experience*

ABOUT THREE YEARS AGO, just as I was completing the last few tests and biopsies for PCD, I spent several days in the hospital due to an infection. My laptop was in its usual place on my blanket, but I was lost in the hyper-alert yet completely unfocused brain haze of the steroid so-lumedrol and too listless to write. A copy of *Breathing for a Living*, cystic fibrosis patient Laura Rothenberg's account of her decision to go on the lung-transplant list and her sub-sequent wait, surgery, and recovery, was on the bedside table. I'd been meaning to read the book for a few weeks but the writing and reading demands of my first semester of graduate school left little time for anything else.

That night, I read the book cover to cover, fully en-grossed in the story of a girl close to my age with experiences that were, on some level, close to mine. I didn't have CF, I wasn't nearly as sick as Laura was, and I certainly wasn't facing a decision as monumental as a double lung transplant. But I *was* in my early twenties, in the hospital, and sick of being sick. In that sense, my feelings were fairly universal. To read about someone else's struggle for air, someone else's cough that wouldn't abate, someone else's frustration with the mood swings, bloating, and muscle cramps that come with steroids—in the midst of the many emotions I experienced reading the book, these similarities somehow comforted me a bit.

I'm not the only one feeling this way.

The first time we met, Brian asked me if I knew anyone else who had PCD. He had no way of knowing how such a natural and innocuous question would have such a complicated truth. After all, for two decades most of my doctors hadn't even seen someone like me. So few people have PCD, or are aware they have it, that the odds of connecting in person are exceedingly slim, a fact of life for many people with rare diseases. Even if I'd been diagnosed earlier in life, I doubt things would be much different.

Brian's experience was the exact opposite. He'd grown up with a definitive diagnosis of cystic fibrosis, and he'd grown up fully entrenched in a community of pediatric patients just like him. He likened his extended hospital stays as a child to "summer camp"—each time he returned, he got to pick up with his hospital friends right where they'd left off. Their CF bond was immediate and impenetrable. They played practical jokes on the nurses on the ward, they immersed themselves in video games, they acted like the typical mischievous children they were. They took the same medications for the same infections, and they passed on intricate knowledge about their diseases to each other. The older patients, the teenagers, were the ones with the most power: they had more illness experience and more life experience, and as such, they served as fairly accurate predictors of what younger patients like Brian would likely face.

The more Brian described his childhood hospital, New York Presbyterian, the more familiar the names and the anecdotes sounded. True, most people with CF his age (twenty-five) would describe similar experiences—only in the past few years have doctors started discouraging groups of patients from congregating because of the communicable diseases they can spread—but there was something specific about his story that gave me pause. It was the depiction of Rothenberg's fellow CF patients that stuck out in my mind even three years later as Brian and I spoke.

As it turns out, Brian knew Laura and had been in the same hospital; they had both described the same cast of characters. He then grew up and began to watch some of his friends die. The fact that he barely knows anyone with CF these days is partially pragmatic: he's since moved away from New York, and though people with CF are living longer than ever before, by his late teens and early twenties, those he'd known with more severe cases had already died. But this lack of community also speaks to his status as a veteran in a different way. He's lived with this disease his entire life, he's watched its life cycle, and he doesn't have many unanswered questions left at this point. What can he learn from patients that he doesn't already know?

I realized when I reflected on Brian's experience that community brings with it the burden of reality. But with it also comes something precious, something that in all those years of misdiagnoses I had never known: shared experience.

When I was finally diagnosed, it was very important to me to find other people with my problems. Determined to find a community, however remote or far-flung it was, I scoured the

Internet looking for PCD and bronchiectasis Web rings and Internet groups. I read all the discussion forum threads in earnest, and even posted now and again. Story after story dealt with misdiagnosis, and our narratives included many of the same details. *This is like reading my life story*, I thought over and over, a virtual approximation of the type of connection Brian must have felt as a child.

To say that diagnosis was the crucial turning point is both obvious and deceiving in its simplicity. It wasn't just that I finally knew what community I belonged to; I could also divide my life into some sort of "before" and "after," a place where all the unlike pieces finally fit together as a seamless whole. Now I could ask other people with PCD and bronchiectasis all the questions I'd compiled. What antibiotics did they take? Did they find chest PT as helpful as I did? Would I be able to have children? Would these diseases shorten my life span? I wanted information stripped bare of medical jargon and technicalities. I'd spent twenty-odd years conversing in that language, and it had never once captured my experiences with illness.

This process of diagnosis, discovery, and initiation cuts across all sorts of age and disease differentials. The proliferation of Web forums and discussion boards and medical blogs all speak to our inherent desire to seek out those like us, to affirm the symptoms and aberrations we've finally found a name for, to assimilate into a community when we've felt isolated from the larger world of the healthy for so long. In fact, Kerri started her diabetes blog, Six Until Me, because whenever she typed "diabetes" into a search engine, all the results she got were heavy on medical terms and reflected very little about the patient experience living with the disease. Now the online diabetes community is thriving globally, spurred on by the simple desire to feel understood.

I find the reverse relationship between illness and community that Brian and I share especially interesting because such a reversal blurs the line between the two dominant types of younger adult patients: those with serious childhood illnesses who are living longer than ever before and those whose autoimmune disorders and other conditions only begin to manifest when they are adults. I hadn't considered how malleable our bond with this type of institutional knowledge is, how the patient community itself is stable, and our needs and expectations are what define and change its role in our lives. Brian may be inching away from the community that so deeply influenced his upbringing just as I am embracing my own communities for the first time, but the stored wisdom and camaraderie of this notion of community health remains accessible.

PART 2

Public Life: Chronic Illness in
an Otherwise Healthy World

15.

REENTRY

*Sometimes the hardest part of
hospitalizations is reentering the
outside world*

W HEN I WAS IN COLLEGE, the hardest part of my numerous hospital stays was often my eventual discharge, the process I have dubbed "reentry." Considering that I hated the Mission: SPACE ride at Disney's Epcot precisely because of the terrifying feeling of being hurtled into an environment that overwhelmed me, this isn't too surprising. But far more disorienting than any ride was the real-life extreme shift between the world of illness and hospitals and the world of the healthy. It jarred me no matter how many times I had to do it. Since reentry will exist as long as there are symptoms that require hospitalizations, it is essential to understand not only why it happens but also how to lessen its impact. Reentry is also the natural place to begin exploring illness in the public sphere, since very often the bustling world we encounter as soon as we leave the hospital doors is the same one least equipped to have us.

My sharpest image of reentry was a sunny spring afternoon during my sophomore year of college. My good friend Jason came to carry my bag and help me make the short journey from the hospital to my campus apartment, which I had been able to see from my hospital room. A few days into my stay, I had the nurse draw the blinds, cutting off my view altogether and placing a literal barrier between the two worlds. Immediately I felt more relaxed; the daytime bustle outside, the pedestrian traffic and shouts and conversations of students, had unnerved me. It reminded me that I was supposed to be out there instead of tethered to my IV pole in a hospital bed and reminded me that soon I would have to find my way back into that throng of motion and progress—after all, hospitals were the places where time stood still.

As Jason and I made our way across the parking lot, the sunlight was too brash, and just opening my eyes seemed to hurt. It was spring, and everything appeared to have come alive while I was in the hospital. The air was thick with the sweet, heady scent of the blossoms on the trees. The lunchtime rush had just ended, and throngs of students poured out of the cafeteria doors, some scurrying across our path on their way to classes, others meandering off in the other direction as they headed to their off-campus houses. The whole scene exhausted me. Even with Jason at my side, I felt incredibly alone.

There are obvious, tangible reasons why prolonged hospitalizations are a huge disruption for anyone: classes or jobs missed, deadlines not met, social functions not attended, plus all the time it takes to put those pieces back together. But more than anything, I hated hospitalizations for the emotional upheavals they caused. The older I got and the more defined I was by commitments and certain roles, the more difficult this transition was for me.

In some ways, prolonged hospitalizations made me less strong, less generous, less compassionate—not the other way around. They created a disconnect between me and anyone else who was not in a hospital, and if I wasn't careful, that chasm could envelop me and almost everyone else who mattered to me. There were the cafeteria lunches or crowded house parties where I drifted out of conversations and just stared at everyone around me: the girls flirting by the frozen-yogurt machine and the guys loudly discussing last night's basketball game, the congested lines forming around the keg in someone's living room or the elaborate process of getting ready to go out on a Friday night. I'd stop, paralyzed by the feeling that while I was around these people, I wasn't one of them. *How can things as trivial as which shoes to wear or who's going to what bar matter?* I'd think. *How can I relate to these people anymore?*

My reactions might seem condescending and self-righteous, and I suppose they were, but sadness is what I felt most during those moments. In reality, I too was often consumed with the same minor worries as my college peers. It's just that being in the hospital took me away from that state of mind, suspended me in a place where I couldn't relate to anyone else. I was on the outside looking in on my own life.

Whether you've been homebound for an extended period of time or are constantly in and out of the hospital, it is inevitable you will experience this clash in cosmos to some degree. In the end, I always managed to complete the process of reentry, even if some attempts took longer than others. So what is essential to transitioning successfully?

What steps do you need to take so you too aren't standing paralyzed in a hospital parking lot, willing the active world around you to freeze just so you catch your breath?

I allowed myself to process those feelings of resentment and to grieve over losses I attributed to being sidelined. It was okay to be anxious and frustrated when I stood on the threshold of returning, but I couldn't let my feelings stop me right in the middle. I realized that, yes, very few people would understand what I'd experienced, but I didn't *need* them to do that. This realization made a huge difference. The healthy were firmly planted on this side of this great divide, and that's exactly where they had to be. They needed to keep living and moving without me so that when I was recovered both physically and emotionally, I had something to move toward. If the cocoon of the hospital comforted me when I could only imagine inertia, than I needed the flurry of resuming my former life to propel me. I needed the thrust of reentry; I just needed to see that it wasn't so terrifying after all.

16.

WHY I DRESS IN LAYERS . . . AND OTHER TALES OF EMBARRASSING INSECURITIES

*Don't waste time thinking people
notice—or care—if you're sick*

No MATTER WHAT OUR AILMENTS ARE, we all have certain signs and symptoms of illness that give us away. It could be the discreet bulge of an insulin pump, the crooked gait of multiple sclerosis, or the stiff, labored movements of arthritis, but certain details reveal our medical information whether we're comfortable with that or not. Over the years, I often went to ridiculous lengths to avoid "looking sick" or standing out in a crowd. The real question, then, is when does what we do to look healthy for others actually become unhealthy for us?

I worried that people who didn't know why I was winded, or why I couldn't carry my bags up the hill, or why my muscles were so weak on certain days that I had to take the escalator would think I was lazy or weak. In thinking this I assumed they even noticed or cared—both of which were unlikely—but this just shows how hypersensitive we can be to our own abnormalities. I also worried about what people who knew I was ill would think if they saw me sweaty from a workout—I imagined they thought I shouldn't have been able to work out, even though doctors encouraged it to "keep things moving" in my lungs. I felt I was making a liar out of myself. The frustrating part of my existence was that I did not—and still do not—fit neatly into categories of wellness or illness, diagnosis or treatment.

I used to wear long sleeves when it was warm outside to cover the deep, ugly IV bruises from hospitalizations. I often wore short sleeves when it was cold, always hoping I could blame it on the heat being turned up too high or having forgotten my sweater, because the steroids I took for my lungs put me in homeostatic haywire and I was always hot or sweaty whenever I was not shivering with cold. I wore foundation to cover up the abnormally flushed cheeks some of my medicines gave me so that, ironically enough, all that was left was a "healthy glow." I can't help but think of Susan Sontag's *Illness as Metaphor*, in which she describes how people grew to consider the rosy glow of TB patients and their gradual wasting away a romantic ideal of beauty and creative spirits. In doing so, society took away from these patients their experience of being sick, replacing the physical realities of illness with a psychological and intellectual ideal.

Perhaps a small part of me wanted to keep up the illusion that I was not so different from everyone else, to ensure there was still a tiny outlet where people did not know I was sick and I could suspend my reality for even a few minutes. It's the central contradiction of illness in the public world, this desire to uphold the identity of a healthy person while still remaining conscious of what will always differentiate us.

The greatest irony in all of this was that I spent so much energy covering up the little signs of illness when the big ones were things I could never hide from friends, classmates, colleagues, or strangers. In college, when I was carried by stretcher from my dorm room to an ambulance just as dinnertime ended and students were pouring out of the dining hall and back into the dorm, there was no way to hide the fact that something was wrong. When I slowly dragged myself from my apartment to the subway stop at rush hour during an acute bout of adrenalitis, my legs so heavy and lethargic I could barely move them, it was patently obvious I wasn't like all the other young professionals whizzing by me. There was no buffer, no distraction or disguise, from my conditions. The painstaking ways I tried to hide the everyday details were my attempt to exert control in whatever smaller ways I could, of evening the score between what made me sick and what made me *me*. I couldn't rewind the episode with the stretcher in my dorm, but I could certainly hide in the bathroom to catch my breath before class started so none of my peers would know I was wheezing from the combination of humid weather and lots of stairs to climb.

Eventually, though, I started to get over it. If a neighbor knocked after hearing me cough, I thanked him for his concern. If my arms were covered in bruises, I wore whatever I wanted anyway. If people stared when I entered the ER gasping for air, I dismissed their gaze. This unencumbered attitude was partially pragmatic, even inevitable: the older I got, the more symptoms and conditions I had to manage. I simply didn't have the time or the inclination to bother juggling all those pretenses, something those of you who also juggle multiple conditions can relate to easily.

But there was more to this maturation than pragmatism, since that implies mere acquiescence. It took me a long time to realize how deeply imbedded the issue of control was in all of this, and it went far beyond the many machinations I went through to hide signs of illness. In spending so much time reacting to the details I thought other people would notice or care about, I was giving them the unwitting power to define me by my illnesses. I made an active decision not to allow the potential perceptions of others to control me. If you give people that ability, then you have ceded your own capacity for self-definition. What I should have been concerned with was the fact that all the outward signs and symptoms in the world didn't determine who I am—but how I responded to them certainly did. It isn't an issue of standing out or "looking sick." The true test of power and security is when we can show perceived weaknesses and define ourselves by our ability to look past them.

17.

"INVISIBLE" ILLNESSES UNMASKED

*When confronted with
misconceptions, consider the source*

B<small>UT YOU DON'T LOOK SICK!</small>"
How many times have you heard that and felt sheer exasperation? It's a known fact that a lot of people only consider illnesses they can "see" as real. Having chronic illness is difficult enough without the added expectation that in order to *be* sick, we should *look* sick, as if the absence of obvious physical manifestations negates the existence of illness.

The pressure of what it means to look sick to healthy people is so pervasive that sometimes it puts us on the defensive. Consider the following scene: It was a weekday morning, and Vicki was at home waiting for the plumbers to come investigate a leak. By all accounts, it was a normal day: she started her morning with chest physiotherapy, worked in her regular nebulizer treatments and medications, and balanced resting with spending time with her infant son. When the doorbell rang and she let the plumbers in, she thought about how the situation must appear to them.

"I was so embarrassed they saw me at home, not working and with a nanny," she says. "I mean, what must they have been thinking? A woman's home all day and still needs help looking after her own child?"

The plumbers didn't comment on any of this or ask questions, but since Vicki didn't "look" sick—though she was extremely thin and her cough would have given her away in due time, she wasn't on oxygen and had no visible signs of trauma or injury—she imagined they were judging her.

"I'm on the lung transplant list," she blurted out to them by way of explanation. Dumbfounded, the men fumbled their expressions of concern and hopes that everything worked out for her, a reaction Vicki finds increasingly common.

"As Dan [her husband] and I share our CF-transplant story with family and friends—and now it's in three local articles—we're finding that a few people ask a ton of questions, but most don't know what to say except that I'm pretty and seem to have a nice family. That's what they notice because I don't look sick in my picture," she says.

Perhaps Vicki overreacted to the perceived judgment she felt from the plumbers—what if they didn't think twice about her being at home?—but her instinct to explain or justify herself to healthy people who don't know she is sick is certainly understandable. It's a frustrating dilemma: We don't want every stranger and passerby to know the intimate details of our lives and often take great pains to keep illness hidden. At the same time, though, we want people to understand why we're not working or why we need a handicapped placard even if we're not in a wheelchair—we don't want to be perceived as lazy, weak, or pampered. I don't need to explain I am sick when I'm being wheeled onto an ambulance, placed in a trauma room, or hooked up to heart monitors; it's when I am not in obvious patient mode that I feel a push and pull between looking healthy and feeling terrible. Similarly, when Vicki does errands with her son and can no longer hold him, she is much more self-conscious of these more public limitations than, say, when she is in the hospital undergoing IV antibiotic treatment. She's expected to be sick as a hospital patient, but as a young, attractive mother with a baby, she is not expected to be weak or to need assistance doing otherwise menial tasks.

Just as there's the expectation that patients should appear a certain way, we have certain expectations about other people. We assume they are judging us and we hope that when we explain our situations it will make a difference—neither of which is always the case. The key is to distinguish between those we'd *like* to understand us better and those we *need* to understand us better. After all, we only have so much energy and inclination to expend eliminating the ignorance of others.

The "invisible illness" phenomenon is one Jenni knows well. Not surprisingly, the same kinds of assumptions about age and constitution that dogged her attempts at getting accurate diagnoses also play a role in her ability to integrate illness into her more public life. "When you look that healthy, there's no visual cue to tell people 'I don't feel well,'" Jenni says. Obviously we shouldn't need to provide other people with visual cues, but part of everyday living dictates that there are situations when we wish we could. Even with her own family Jenni often dealt with misconceptions about her disease. For example, part of her treatment plan involves daily stretching. During a trip home, one of her relatives saw her doing her stretches and said to her, "How come you can't even touch your toes? You're way too young to not be able to touch your toes!"

At the time, Jenni felt hurt and resentful of her relative's implication that she was weak or somehow falling below a preconceived notion of what someone her age should be. "Looking back, I realize he had no idea. He couldn't begin to understand my experience," she says—and he didn't try to understand. That difference is critical. There will always be people who aren't willing to try to learn more about conditions and their implications. Their expectations of us will not change, so what has to happen is that our expectations of others must evolve. You can't persuade or enlighten people who don't choose to listen, so it's not worth feeling you need to justify yourself or your conditions to them. Focus on the friends, family, and interested acquaintances who want to know more, who ask questions or offer support or admit they aren't familiar with your condition but want to be. It's inevitable we will be judged on the basis of "invisible" illnesses, but not every source of criticism deserves or benefits from our attempts at justification or explanation.

"I don't really care that much anymore if people can't understand me, because I don't need them to," Jenni says, grateful for the support of close friends and the community of chronically ill people she's fostered over the years. She's not saying she doesn't need anyone; in fact, she's saying just the opposite: since she has the encouragement and support of the people who matter most, the assumptions and accusations of people who don't want to be educated do not have the power to hurt her.

This same mentality extends to those people who equate being sick with a certain "ideal patient" in mind. They may express skepticism when confronted with people who are diagnosed with chronic fatigue syndrome, fibromyalgia, or chronic headaches or migraines. Responses like "So you're tired, who isn't?" or "Can't you just rest and get over it?" or "Everyone gets headaches, what's the big deal?" are, unfortunately, still part of the public lexicon when it comes to chronic conditions whose origins and manifestations aren't as easily understood. However infuriating and irrational such comments are, they only have the power to define or validate our conditions if we allow that to happen. There are all sorts of reasons why people find it easy to scorn or deny illness, especially in younger people who "should" look and act healthy—fear, ignorance, intolerance, to name some. But other people's attitudes do not validate our conditions.

Just how prevalent is this tendency to ascribe certain physical attributes to the sick? Vicki describes a recent trip to the ER when the man helping transport her from her car into the wheelchair told her she didn't look sick. If being rushed to the emergency room and ushered into a wheelchair aren't signs that someone is unwell, then what are?

At this point, she is used it. "People have their own images of illness, similar to their own images of marriage, divorce, happiness, love, etc. They see what they were raised to see . . . what they know from their own experiences, but not from a broader spectrum," she says.

Her point rings true when it comes to our perspective as patients too. There have been times when I've heard someone cough and thought to myself, "That's not a *real* cough; he must be healthy and just have a cold," or seen otherwise agile-looking patients in the waiting room of a rheumatologist's office and said to myself, "They can't be in that much pain. Look at how quickly they get up out of their seats." I feel guilty when I think this way, because intellectually I know that surface symptoms very often fail to encapsulate the depth of a disease or illness experience. Yet because I know what it is like to cough so hard I cough up blood and because I have watched my mother not even be able to brush her own hair for several years due to her advanced arthritis and degenerative joint disease, I assume people who do not manifest the same traits I know aren't sick. I have my own expectation of what "sick" looks and sounds like, and while my own rubric may be far more nuanced and specific than the average healthy person's, it is still clouded with my own biases and personal history.

Vicki acknowledges doing the same thing. "I see people with CF who are tall and muscular and my first thought is, 'You don't look like you have CF'—probably because I look in the mirror and they don't look like me and the others who are malnourished. I think to myself, 'Are they really that sick?' They are, but again, it's based on my own image of what a sick CFer looks like. I guess we just have to learn not to sweat the small stuff with these things. In the end, it really doesn't matter what other people think. Really, it doesn't," she says.

Regardless of our specific conditions, at some point we will all face awkward exchanges with people who come to our houses, people who see us in grocery stores or shopping malls, or even other patients whose appearance somehow casts doubt on our own conceptions of illness. Everyone has an opinion, but that doesn't mean we should allow their opinions to invalidate our realities.

18.
THE PATIENT TRANSLATOR

Explaining rare diseases is an
exercise in precision and patience

PRIMARY CILIARY DYSKINESIA. Pri•mar•y cil•i•ar•y dys•ki•nes•i•a.

It doesn't exactly roll off the tongue, does it?

I refer to it in passing as PCD, but with limited success. Since no one knows what the letters stand for and we're living in the MySpace age, I fear the first association people make with the abbreviation is the Pussycat Dolls, the all-girls' band. The same thing happens when I say I have bronchiectasis; more often than not, even when I'm talking to a nurse in the ER, people assume I must actually mean "bronchitis" and just forgot how to pronounce it correctly.

As anyone with a rare or little-known disease can attest, explaining what is wrong to people who have no clue what we're talking about or no context for our problems is challenging. My PCD is never going to have the cache of more common diseases, just like Angela's Ehlers-Danlos syndrome or my father's polymyositis are never going to spark nods of recognition or be featured in television commercials or glossy magazines. As a result, we're often thrust into the role of translator, responsible for conveying unfamiliar information in familiar terms, and our ability to do that is one of the most important tools we can have in our repertoire.

I don't care if people can't spell or say my conditions correctly—to be honest, I'm not even sure my own siblings could tell you what "PCD" stands for if put to the test, but they know what living with it is like, and that's what's important. However, when I'm rushed to the hospital and I'm met with blank stares when I say what I have, I do worry because that has very real implications for my treatment. If seasoned hospital staff sometimes do not recognize or understand my conditions, how can I expect the average person to? It's not as if I am constantly in situations where I need people to understand, obviously, but sometimes being what a friend of mine calls "clinically interesting" can be isolating.

Officially, a rare, or "orphan," disease is one that affects fewer than two hundred thousand people nationwide. The National Organization for Rare Disorders estimates that some six thousand rare diseases collectively affect more than twenty-five million Americans.[1] That's a whole lot of mangled spellings, garbled pronunciations, and question marks. Consider the fact that the list of those six thousand diseases does not even list bronchiectasis among them (though I did let out a little cheer that PCD, Ehlers-Danlos syndrome, and polymyositis were there) and you start to grasp the true enormity of the rare disease population.

Any medical personnel or EMT crew member knows the standard operating procedure for dealing with a diabetic high or low or an asthma attack in a known asthma patient, for example, because these are diseases that affect millions of people and are ones they confront frequently. Even non-medical people often have *some* inkling that diabetics worry about blood sugar and what foods they eat, or know that an asthmatic often uses an inhaler during an attack. But for those of us blessed with chronic conditions that also happen to be rare, it's not often we experience any semblance of familiarity or understanding.

Far more troublesome and isolating than when people do not recognize rare diseases is when their only understanding of them is inaccurate. It is an innately human tendency to fear or dislike what we don't understand. In his classic 1932 film *Freaks*, Tod Browning explores the types of misinformation and misrepresentation that leads our society to view physical deformities as "freakish." More than seventy years later, in 2006, patients and advocacy groups were enraged by the way EDS was portrayed on ABC's *Medical Mysteries* show, making a mockery of the realities of the disease. Since most people wouldn't have even heard of EDS until the show aired, the skewed representation of the disease was even more damaging.

Navigating translation issues with rare diseases is a process of discernment. I don't owe the average person who looks askance at me after a coughing bout an explanation any more than Angela owes the passersby who ask how she dislocated her shoulder the truth about her disease or my father owes the golfers who wonder why he can only attempt to play if he uses a golf cart an explanation of why his muscles are so weak and he tires so easily.

But what about friends and acquaintances, people who have at least some degree of vested interest in our health status but may not be fluent in medical jargon? Even if people

I come into contact with regularly know I don't cough simply because I have a cold or I don't wheeze because I have asthma, does that mean "primary ciliary dyskinesia" or "bronchiectasis" will mean anything to them? Probably not, and I don't need it to. If people in work or social settings ask me for more details, I usually say something like "I have respiratory diseases that prevent me from clearing infections in my lungs." If they've heard of cystic fibrosis—interestingly, I find many people have—then I'll take it a step further: "It's similar to CF in terms of the coughing and the mucus production and is treated in similar ways, though it's caused by different things," I'll say, and leave it at that. I try to put it in simple terms that are still authentic to my experience without being overwhelming. When possible, I relate it to symptoms or conditions people are more familiar with, because familiarity breeds comfort and confidence. After all this time, I've learned that I don't need people to understand the intricacies of my illness—but I do want them to be informed enough to abandon their fears I am a harbinger of infectious disease. Beyond that, I'm content to cough away without compunction.

19.
ANOTHER KIND OF MEDICAL STUDENT

*Achieving success in higher
education takes a different type of
intelligence*

WHEN I READ RECENTLY that DePaul University in
Chicago launched the Chronic Illness Initiative
(CII) to provide support for chronically ill students, I was
elated, relieved, and a bit surprised. I hadn't expected academia to catch up to what is very clearly an emerging trend
in higher education so soon. Given that upward of six hundred thousand chronically ill adults turn eighteen each
year[1] and many of them will go on to matriculate in institu-
tions of higher education, it's clear that this population deserves recognition and accommodation. DePaul's School
for New Learning, under whose auspices the CII operates,
posits a blessedly logical explanation for the program:

"Students who struggle with illnesses that unpredictably
increase and decrease in severity such as chronic fatigue

syndrome, rheumatoid arthritis, lupus or illnesses with frequent hospitalizations such as cancer or heart disease, may have found it difficult, if not impossible, to meet the requirements of a conventional college program."[2]

Often if colleges have any programs or resources to support chronically ill students, they are lumped together with those resources and programs set up for students with learning disabilities. Both groups deserve time, attention, and support, but each group's needs are vastly different. More than anything else, chronically ill students need flexibility with deadlines, course loads, and expectations when their conditions flare or unexpected medical crises occur, and it is difficult to find that in a traditional undergraduate program. This unpredictability of chronic illness is especially challenging; professors don't like it when students don't show up for weeks, particularly if they don't really understand why.

"Faculty generally don't know what to do with chronically ill students or what standards to apply to them," says CII director Lynn Royster, J.D., Ph.D. Her impetus for the program came from watching her previously academically strong son struggle with his grades when he became chronically ill. Serving as a liaison between faculty and students to help bridge the understanding gap is one of the more significant features of the program, along with educating professors about the waxing and waning nature of chronic illness—something distinctly different from the physically disabled students universities are more used to accommodating.

"It doesn't matter how fast students complete the program. What's more important is that they meet success and stay well," says Paula Kravitz, MSW, who works with students in the CII and advises them on course loads and schedules. There is no time limit on how long it takes to earn a degree, and students can take as many or as few classes a semester as they see fit (though this does not preclude certain financial aid requirements). She emphasizes the program allows students to individually plan how to be successful. For some, this means taking courses during the summer and fall and avoiding taking a lot of winter classes if they know their fibromyalgia pain or chronic fatigue symptoms are worse when it's cold. For others, online courses in which they can telecommute from different parts of the country and don't have to leave their doctors and hospitals makes a lot of sense too. Among other developments, the program also runs an online discussion forum for students and is gathering data to pursue further research on chronic illness.

"Just our being there validates the students' sense of self. They know that there are people who believe they are capable even though they are sick," says Royster.

As a college student living with chronic pancreatitis, Jade Cooper has experienced many of the obstacles Royster and Kravitz mention, and has also been the recipient of the kind of support so necessary to survive higher education. When she was a freshman at Texas Tech University, she was hospitalized for almost two weeks—the period in which she finally received her diagnosis—and fell behind in her classes. She could only drop four classes over the course of her college career, and knowing the strong likelihood she would have severe flares again, she didn't want to drop most of them as a freshman. Since she was too far behind to catch up in all those courses, she decided to withdraw from school altogether and wasn't able to enroll again until the following fall. Having the flexibility to alter her schedule and set her own pace would have minimized such a major disruption to her academic career and would have made taking care of her health needs easier.

Ultimately, Jade transferred to South Plains College, a much smaller school where she could better manage her stress level and her chronic pain. A special services program at her school documents her medical condition and educates her professors about her absences and the particular complications her condition causes. "Sometimes even when I am in class, I'm really not there because the drugs make it so hard to think," she says. Having a liaison to help her professors understand this side effect of the pain medication she needs to take during acute flares makes a big difference. Were she to appear healthy and be able to attend most classes, her teachers might attribute any difficulty she experienced to laziness or incompetence, rather than the effect of strong pain medicine.

Even in the absence of institutionalized support like what Jade has and the CII offers its students, there are still ways for chronically ill students to find success in the classroom. Consistent communication, proactive planning, and understanding the knowledge base of faculty and administrators are the most important tools in terms of integrating chronic illness in the classroom, and they are all things that can be attained by individual students.

I had a lifetime of being a sick student to prepare me for college, and I took the mistakes and hard-earned lessons with me. Like so many students with childhood illness, I missed days, sometimes weeks, of grammar school for various infections and surgeries. I'd been conditioned to view the school year as a cycle of makeup work. I'd catch up, then miss more, make up the work on my own, and then get sick again. This cycle was magnified in high school, because in addition to nine academic classes a day, a host of extracurricular activities, and my "usual" illnesses, I contracted mono that lasted nineteen months and developed into chronic fatigue syndrome (CFS). At the worst point during my junior year, I slept twenty hours a day and didn't go to school for two solid months. At more manageable points of my junior and senior years, I made it in for a few half days a week and made up all the work I missed at home whenever I felt up to it.

My high school years were incredibly stressful due to my illnesses. There were lots of parent conferences to explain why I couldn't always hand something in the day it was due but that I would turn it in, why I couldn't always schedule a makeup lab session at seven thirty A.M., why I could be there one day and not be able to attend the next. I wish I'd thought to sit down with each individual teacher and make decisions about priorities—which "busywork" assignments I could skip to focus on the papers, tests, and quizzes; which classroom activities didn't necessarily need to be replicated on my own when I had mountains of other work to wade through. It's something I always make sure to do with my own college writing students who have chronic illnesses. We decide which assignments are crucial to them passing the course and which ones are expendable.

Some of the stress I experienced in high school was of my own doing. I wouldn't entertain dropping down to less rigorous sections or taking a leave of absence to recuperate and then repeat my junior year. I put an immense amount of pressure on myself to get As in every class, on every assignment. I graduated as covaledictorian, but at an enormous cost to myself and my health. I wish I'd known then that in the real world, none of that mattered. No one cares if you were first in your class—I can't even imagine a situation in which that would come up now. They care if you can perform your job well, if you are articulate, if you have integrity and self-awareness.

Still, it was never really about the grades for me in high school. It was about losses—loss of my social life, loss of positions like editor in chief of the school paper when I had to resign, loss of my identity as anything other than a sick girl. I think my family and friends understood the social ramifications of chronic illness, how isolating it was to go weeks without seeing friends, without lunchtime chats and after-school activities. I'm not sure many of them understood how crucial the identity of a student was to me, how deeply I connected my success in the classroom to my sense of worth. My grades and my academic standing were all I had left to define me, and I wasn't going to lose anything else to illness.

I went into my freshman year of college knowing I needed to be proactive about managing school and chronic illness—good thing, because while my CFS flares were much less severe, my lungs deteriorated with each passing semester. In fact, I'd never been sicker. I took four classes my freshman fall instead of the standard five, which was still enough credit for me to remain a full-time student. I also took evening courses during the summer that counted toward my graduation requirements. This gave me some leeway during the regular semester in case I did need to withdraw from a course. I spent several weeks in the hospital early one spring semester, and when my dean suggested I withdraw from a course to lighten my load and makeup work, I was relieved I had the summer credits behind me to do so without delaying my graduation.

More than anything, I tried to communicate with and to educate my professors. I'd linger after the first class of each semester and briefly explain my conditions and how unpredictable they could be. I assured them that I could provide medical documentation and that if I missed class, I would get the lecture notes from my peers. I had compassionate, understanding professors who allowed me the flexibility to make up missed work without further risking my health. I also had the guidance of a wise dean who wanted me to succeed personally and academically. Make no mistake about it, I never would have been able to graduate on time and with a GPA I was proud of were it not for the educators who believed in my ability to do the work and didn't mind if it was a little bit late.

But I also think they were willing to extend the occasional deadline and remain flexible with me because I was diligent and stayed on top of things—I e-mailed papers from my hospital bed and studied for finals hooked up to oxygen, and I always made sure I notified the appropriate people when I faced longer hospitalizations. I understood that extenuating circumstances didn't excuse me from doing the work, and they understood that extenuating circumstances sometimes meant I couldn't be there in person. I still had a lot of growing up to do in terms of realizing my limitations and taking on too many social and extracurricular activities, but in terms of the classroom experience, I had found a way to thrive and an environment in which to do so. I'd been a sick student for enough years to know that the more people understand and are kept informed, the more they are able to do for me. In what amounted to a "Freaky Friday" moment, I found myself telling one of my students the exact same thing—that the more I knew about his illness and the more documentation I had, the more flexible and accommodating I could be.

If classroom success is so dependent on a mutual understanding and open communication, what happens when that breaks down? Just as my lung problems worsened by the time I was in college and I was a lot sicker, Angela's EDS symptoms are much more pronounced now that she is in college, and it has had a profound impact on her experience. Part of it can be explained away by disease progression; her joints were simply more stable when she was younger. But she also underestimated the amount of medical problems she would have, an understandable outcome when you're talking about a chronic condition like EDS. At the same time her dislocations and surgeries increased, so too did her course load and other responsibilities. Something had to give, and when her EDS landed her in the hospital, it was school that suffered.

"Working full time didn't help either. I started out in an accelerated degree program, and when I failed to keep up and maintain the minimum GPA, I felt a lot of pressure to at least graduate in four years. That didn't happen either. I'll have my bachelor's degree in a couple months, five years after matriculating. Had I taken a more manageable course load, without worrying about finishing on time, I would not have had to repeat so many courses, and even if I wouldn't have finished any sooner, I would have finished with a much better GPA," she says.

So she was sicker than she expected and took on a schedule that was too jam-packed to allow for illness. She's certainly not the only one to do that—in fact, expecting too much of our bodies and giving them too little downtime to recover is a common refrain among patients.

"My high school teachers were much more flexible," says Angela, "when it came to giving makeup exams and accepting late assignments—which was basically only an issue when I had to have surgery." Her college experiences, however, include the following scenarios: taking makeup exams that were harder than the original, having her grade calculated on a different scale from the rest of her peers, and being penalized for missing in-class activities and lectures even if she could make up the work on her own. Having a rare disease like EDS doesn't help the situation—if nurses in her local ER still react skeptically to her, imagine how hard it must be to try to explain it to a professor with no working medical knowledge.

"In cases where I've had ER documentation to explain my absence from an exam, the nature of my disorder was never an issue. However, when I miss lectures, quizzes, exams because of a dislocation or subluxation that I've fixed myself and therefore have no medical documentation for— as is usually the case—I'm faced with the task of providing an explanation. I've had more than one professor respond by telling me that I don't belong in college. Others have suggested I withdraw from the university until I'm 'better,' " she says.

As a patient, I am enraged by this type of comment. As a college instructor, I'm immensely disappointed by it. As much as I tout the value of communication and educating professors and administrators, this only works when the intended audience has enough respect to try to learn.

20.

FULL DISCLOSURE: HOW MUCH DO HEALTHY PEOPLE NEED TO KNOW?

*Knowing how to disclose illness in
the workplace is just as important as
knowing when to do so*

WHEN YOU'RE IN SCHOOL, no one else is impacted by your absence if you don't feel well and miss a lecture. It's completely different in the world of work, however. If you don't show up, your absence affects everyone else who depends on you.

Illness does not defer to time stamps, meetings, or class schedules. What's even more challenging than hiding the physical symptoms of illness is deciding what to do when those symptoms pose potential problems in our work environment. From the fear of losing a job or facing stigmatization by colleagues or superiors to the notion that illness is supremely personal and should remain outside a professional environment, the decision about when and if to disclose conditions in the workplace is a loaded one.

Rosalind Joffe, a career coach specializing in working with executives with chronic illness, sees balancing the equally important roles of patient and employee as one of the most significant issues facing the workplace today. She was diagnosed with autoimmune diseases—multiple sclerosis and ulcerative colitis—as a younger woman in the midst of building a career and a family, so she's faced the same types of situations as her clients. Emphasizing a point at the core of much of this book, she points out that more young people are living longer with serious chronic diseases and are living far more "normalized" lives than ever before, meaning they are entering and remaining in a workforce that, for the most part, isn't equipped to deal with them on an individual or institutionalized scale yet.

"Few organizations are paying attention to this because most chronic illnesses are invisible and people tend to hide their illnesses," Joffe says. This can cause problems not only in terms of job function but also job satisfaction. Research shows people are more successful when they have a supportive boss and tend to be happier when they have at least a few people at work with whom they have closer, more personal relationships—and they tend to feel even more isolated and disconnected by illness when no one knows what's going on with their health.

So where do you draw the line between what healthy people need to know about your health and what you can keep to yourself?

The environments in multinational companies, small businesses, and in retail, research, and academic settings are all different, as are the relationships patient-employees have with co-workers and superiors, so there is a lot of room for variation in terms of when and how to disclose illness. Those conditions notwithstanding, Joffe offers a bottom line for all patients to consider, regardless of our chosen professions or our degree of reluctance to divulge personal details: "The point where you *have* to disclose is when your illness starts to get in the way of your ability to perform your job and the quality of that performance," she says. "If you can't do the job as is expected, then you have to figure out what you need in order to do it, if that's possible, and then you have to ask for accommodations." If your health problems don't directly impact your ability to do the job— if you're an arthritic whose flares are infrequent and not severe or a Crohn's patient whose symptoms respond well to treatment and largely subside, for example—then you don't have to disclose.

This is, of course, a minimum standard. You may still *choose* to tell certain people, but the imperative isn't quite the same. Kerri, who works for dLife, a diabetes media company, has no reason to hide her type 1 diabetes status— after all, one of her job requirements is to write a column about living with the disease. If there's a corporate culture assimilated to insulin pumps and testing blood sugar, it's hers. Brian is a research analyst for a vendor for pharmaceutical companies, and the atmosphere there is obviously different from Kerri's workplace. Though some people may have feared "scaring off" employers by doing so, he disclosed his CF status during his first interview and was still hired anyway, a sign that they understood enough about the disease to know he would still be able to perform the job. Brian's decision to be so forthright from the outset mirrors my own decision to alert my superiors: our disclosures had less to do with immediate concerns about productivity but instead took into account the *potential* for hospitalizations or unexpected sick days, disruptions that could temporarily impede our job performance but did not affect our overall capabilities.

Sometimes Joffe's bottom line, is, unfortunately, all too easy to identify. When I was in my second year of graduate school, I took a weekend job at the Devon Nicole House (DNH) at Children's Hospital Boston. The DNH offers affordable, flexible accommodations in a community house for the families of pediatric patients, and my job consisted of checking families in and out, helping plan group activities, and lending support to parents and siblings, whether that meant listening to updates about their children or helping them navigate the public transportation system. Two months into it, my adrenal system crashed. Adrenal insufficiency left me with extreme fatigue and muscle weakness so overwhelming that most days I could barely walk. Weekends were especially tough because the whole week's worth of fatigue accumulated. I physically could not get to the DNH, and even if I could, I was not up to being in charge of a houseful of families—I could hardly brush my own teeth. Though it was emotionally painful for me to resign, the decision was, in the end, an easy one to make because there wasn't really much to decide. I simply could not perform the job, and I owed it to my boss to tell her that as soon as possible so she could find someone who could.

Given the range of chronic diseases and the numerous professional environments that exist, such decisions are not usually clear-cut. In terms of teaching, I can't think about my position as a writing instructor without thinking about what I call my "witching hours." For whatever reason, between four and six P.M. are brutal for me—I am much more congested, I wheeze even more audibly, and the color drains from my face just as the dark circles under my eyes come out of hiding. My physical therapist says that my "morning lungs" and my "afternoon lungs" sound like they belong to entirely different people. Since I often teach health professions students, this phenomenon is somewhat more conspicuous—try hiding a "productive" cough from a roomful of nurses or hopeful medical school applicants. On especially bad days, I see the inquisitive looks on their faces. I joke about it with them when they ask if I'm "still sick"—"Must be the plague you people keep passing around to each other," I say—and though there's some truth to that, it's also a way of answering them without disclosing too much. While I bring in my personal experience as a health writer when it's germane to the discussion, I have never felt my personal medical issues are appropriate or relevant to their work, our work.

Yet my conditions also represent a *potential* threat to my ability to do my job. I can't conduct a class if I am unexpectedly in the hospital, and it's not like I can just call in sick and teach an extra class the day I return. These are the types of judgment calls that make disclosure so nuanced and so closely tied to the specific conditions of our jobs. When talking to my superiors, I've chosen to stick to the most basic facts, the ones that impact their time and their ability to satisfy students, without burdening them with the intricacies of diseases they've never heard of before. Typically, I tell them I have chronic respiratory diseases that sometimes flare unexpectedly, and while I don't anticipate many disruptions, I have colleagues who can step in at the last minute if I need them to. I feel it's fair to the department and my students to be proactive about setting up a contingency plan.

Joffe considers these types of discussions action-based: you initially disclose certain facts to change a particular outcome in your workplace. The more ongoing dialogue, one that emphasizes creativity and collaboration when it comes to accommodations, is explored in the following chapter, but this process begins with the conscious decision to reveal debilitating symptoms. First consider if you even want to name the disease or just talk about the symptoms, since that's what is most relevant. Though disclosure may feel like it places patients in a vulnerable position, Joffe maintains that through our presentation of information, we can strongly influence the outcome. She advises her clients to keep their tone matter-of-fact and to provide their bosses or human resources personnel with concrete ways their specific conditions could interfere with their job. "You have to accept that rarely are people going to be able to meet your emotional needs, but if you are clear in your request, they will be more willing and able to help," she says, so the more specific we can be about the relationship between symptoms and productivity, the better.

Another aspect of disclosure Joffe says is particularly sensitive is the reaction colleagues may have once the condition is revealed. Having spent twenty years trying to avoid "looking sick" or letting my patient identity impact my public identity, I can understand this fear well. Who wants to be labeled as the "sick one," especially when the leap from "sick" to "not as productive" or "unreliable" isn't too difficult to make for people who don't understand the nature of chronic illness? There's an underlying potential to associate "sickness" with "weakness" in the public domain, a tendency that is even more pronounced in the workplace. However, Joffe's experience seems to show that people are much less concerned with our health problems than we are. "At a client's request, I've interviewed colleagues about their work performance, and invariably they don't have nearly as many issues with the illness as my client fears," she says, noting that this provides an additional incentive for those patients who may wish to establish more authenticity about their lives with their colleagues.

Assuming a professional or public identity means that, to varying degrees, what we do and how we feel not only affects our ability to do our jobs but also affects all the people whose own jobs are tied up in ours. For some of us, there comes a point when for all our sakes, the fair and responsible thing to do is disclose our health conditions. When we initiate a dialogue, when we're factual, concrete, and maintain confidence in our skills, we can better accommodate our needs.

21.

INTELLIGENT DESIGN

Be creative in adapting careers to
accommodate chronic conditions

WHEN YOU'RE TWENTY-FOUR OR TWENTY-FIVE, what are you if you don't work?"

That was the central question plaguing Vicki when she faced the difficult decision of choosing between her career aspirations and her health. Traditionally, our twenties and thirties constitute the time when we're focused on building a career and establishing networks and experiences that we will carry through most of our lives, and that career is often closely linked to our identities. Think about the typical conversations we have in bars, at cocktail parties, or other places where we're grouped with people we don't know—more often than not, "So, what do you do?" is the first question we turn to after the initial introductions, and there's a reason for that. The workplace isn't just where we get our money or our sense of accomplishment or fulfillment; it's also where we cultivate social relationships and camaraderie.

So what do you do when your health gets in the way of all of that?

The solution is as varied as the experience of living with different illnesses. For some of us, it becomes a question of adapting current jobs to better suit our needs and finding companies and organizations where flexibility and creativity in job design are valued. For others, chronic conditions may necessitate switching career trajectories altogether, negotiating between interests and talents and physical limitations. Depending on the nature of the disease, some of us will also reach the point where we have to remove ourselves from the workplace entirely. No stage in this process is easy or enviable, but the reality is that many of us will have to confront the tension between what we *want* to do and what our bodies *can* do—and a willingness to confront that difficult decision can have a huge impact on the quality of our lives.

Issues of economics and corporate culture aside, the emotional implications of adjusting careers or leaving the workplace are huge. If you are someone who defines yourself by what you do and, inevitably, what you achieve, chronic illness is just as devastating emotionally as it is physically. For Vicki, a well-educated, highly motivated woman who grew up in a family where a hard-driving work ethic was the expected norm and needing to rest was considered a form of weakness, acknowledging the toll her job in executive recruiting was taking on her health was a painful process. By the time the situation escalated to where she was throwing up when she reached the office and experiencing bouts of road rage, she knew she needed to get some help sorting through her emotions and the competing needs of her body and her ambition.

"I was twenty-four . . . twenty-five and in a big depression. I hated my illness and kept trying to deny what was happening," she says. The decision to leave the job she loved was excruciating, but given the disease progression she was experiencing, ultimately she had no choice. Not only could she no longer perform her job, but attempting to do so also seriously undermined her health.

She went to counseling to help her work through the profound loss and deep anger she felt, and it was there that her counselor pointed out something she hadn't realized: "Your life will now become about your relationships with others," she told her. Though it came at a huge emotional and physical expense, her decision to stop working is what allowed her to take care of herself enough so that she was able to nourish and sustain relationships to the people most important to her.

On a smaller level, I can relate to Vicki's sense of loss and anger over all the things illness took away from her. Over the years, I've resigned from so many things on account of my health: positions on school newspapers, permanent freelance jobs I adored, working on an academic journal, my job at the Devon Nicole House. With each resignation and each tortuous explanation I composed in my head, I started to think more and more about my long-term career choices. I didn't want to spend a lifetime having these awkward talks.

After my college graduation and the epiphany that I didn't want to go to law school, I'd cobbled together a variety of jobs: a day job at a major publishing company, a freelance book editing gig at a small business publisher, and other freelance editorial projects. The overwhelming guilt I experienced over missing days of work and the physical toll the long days took on me all conspired to worsen my health and my resistance to infection. This happened before I switched doctors and got correct diagnoses, so I was pretty seriously ill at this time: I had steroid myopathy from all my prednisone that made getting up and down the stairs of my fourth-floor walk-up difficult, and I was frequently in the hospital for respiratory infections. I lived in a state of tension—my lung problems were unpredictable and my status changed fast, making it impossible to guarantee I would be at work every day at eight thirty A.M.

I left work to attend graduate school. Combined with new treatments and increased understanding of my conditions, I began to live less in the extremes of being busy or bed-bound. Like Vicki, my background emphasized hard work and achievement, and it was still difficult sometimes to say no to projects or jobs when I was already busy, but I reminded myself that the more I did to ensure I wasn't so sick that I needed to be hospitalized, the more I could accomplish personally and professionally.

Most of my friends left their respective graduate programs with concrete, "cocktail-party" appropriate jobs—as lawyers, consultants, doctors, nurses. I'd always assumed I would join their ranks, but that wasn't where my interests and my health were leading me. I'd taught undergraduate writing courses while working toward my MFA, and I enjoyed it more than I'd ever thought I would. My students were interesting and motivated, and our classroom discussions were fruitful and productive. There was another great advantage to teaching in higher education: the schedule was more flexible. Rosalind Joffe considers flexibility the most important accommodation for most chronically ill patients, and that makes sense. I could teach a few classes in one day and still have time to make doctor's appointments or get chest PT. I could arrange my schedule so that I had one or two days a week where I could be "down"—even if I was reading student papers all day and night, I could do it from the couch and take breaks when I needed them. Lastly, between school breaks, summer, and the weeks where the essays didn't flood in, I could devote time to my freelance writing.

Whether it translates into working from home a couple of days a week or establishing alternative work hours—arriving later and leaving later, for example—these kinds of creative compromises are typically the most effective way chronically ill workers can still succeed in the workplace. Since self-employment is not feasible or preferable for everyone, there are other steps that can allow you to cater to your illness and still remain productive. However, flexibility entails more than simply arranging different work hours or telecommuting; sometimes patients must think in terms of the types of jobs they perform. Sometimes taking a job in the same field but with different physical demands is the most viable compromise. Joffe relays the experience of a client of hers who worked in research. Logging long hours in the lab exacerbated his physical symptoms of multiple sclerosis, so before he got so sick that he'd have to quit, he transitioned into a project management role. This way, he was still a vital participant in the field he loved, but his participation did not cause his health to deteriorate.

Maintaining a professional identity and sense of purpose is closely tied to quality of life and personal satisfaction. Too often, career success comes at the expense of our health, but it doesn't always have to be that way. Proactive planning and being realistic about your professional goals and individual health needs are essential components of this so-called intelligent design toward chronic illness in the workplace.

22.

FINANCIAL FRICTION

*Flexibility and finances aren't
always mutually compatible, but
some sacrifices and prioritization
are worth the risk*

I'T'S ONE THING TO ADVOCATE for creative solutions to
staying in the workplace despite chronic illness. It's another thing altogether to live with the financial ramifications
of those solutions. But for those people who have traded in
more conventional stability for better health outcomes, the
benefits usually outweigh the very real drawbacks.

The flexibility of my new career came, quite literally, at a
price: adjunct professors are notoriously underpaid, we
don't receive benefits, and there is no chance of promotion
no matter how glowing our evaluations are. Freelancing of
any type has the potential to yield a significant income, but
like with any nascent career, getting to the point where you
can rely on the stability of that income takes a long time.
Still, the risk is worth it to me if it means I am professionally

fulfilled and my quality of life is better, if I am in the hospital less and able to do the things I want to with less disruptions and complications.

At the same time, I cannot just gloss over the fact that I would not have sustainable health insurance as an adjunct and a freelance writer were I not married. My husband's health insurance allows me the luxury of choice, and I know if I had to trade in my unconventional, patchwork method of working full-time for a "normal" full-time job with benefits, I would be much sicker, and my relationships would bear the strain of my health. Though I'll explore the impact of what I call the "chronic income gap" on relationships later in the book, the reality of health insurance is something you cannot disassociate from any pragmatic discussion about illness and the workplace. Many of my adjunct colleagues do not have health insurance, and their solution to this is to "stay healthy," as they say. Clearly this is not an option for anyone with chronic illness.

So often, the choices we know we should make for our bodies' sakes are intertwined in many conflicting variables. Jenni decided to leave her last office job to start her own communications company so she could better manage her health and lifestyle, but it was a choice she would not have made if she wasn't covered by her husband's health insurance. Now that she has founded ChronicBabe, combining her desire to educate and connect young women with chronic illness and her freelance writing experience, the fruits of that creative planning and strategy are readily apparent. Her income isn't yet what it once was, but it has been a sacrifice well worth making in consideration of all the other benefits. She's doing something she loves, something that makes a difference in other people's lives, and her health is also better for it. When she experiences an acute fibromyalgia flare and needs to rest, she knows she has the authority to do that and that she can compensate for missed time when she is up to it.

For twenty-year-old Jade, decisions about what she wants to do when she graduates from college are foremost in her mind and implications of her chronic pancreatitis are at the heart of those decisions. She is covered under her parents' health insurance until she turns twenty-four but is already hoping to secure her own benefits so she can remain fully in charge of her health care needs. "Having chronic illness means there is no way around health insurance—situations are always going to arise where you're going to need it. That's just the way it is," she says. She used to work in a restaurant, but the long hours spent on her feet left her little time to rest or rejuvenate, and her health suffered for it. She's given up her previous goal of entering the restaurant and hotel management profession precisely because of the physical toll such jobs exact, but it wasn't an easy decision. She now works part-time at a bank and hopes to attain full-time employment with benefits in banking.

One obvious ramification of needing to work in certain jobs just for the benefits is the physical toll on a patient's health. But there's an equally compelling consequence, a phenomenon dubbed "health-insurance-related job lock"—not only does your health suffer, but your job progression and employee satisfaction can also stagnate if you feel you can't leave a certain job because you'll lose the benefits. Research published in the *Journal of Policy Analysis and Management* suggests that more than 64 percent of nonelderly Americans who are insured get that insurance from their employer; thus the relationship between insurance coverage and job mobility is a significant one.[1] Unlike previous studies of job mobility that failed to isolate workers with chronic illness or family members with chronic illness, this research found that for the sample of workers who depended on their employer for insurance, "chronic illness reduced job mobility by about 40 percent as compared with otherwise similar workers who did not rely on their employer for coverage."[2]

What do you do if you're one of those patients who, whether it's due to health insurance job lock or the fact that you aren't interested or able to start your own company, feels you must remain in the mainstream corporate environment? Again, getting results requires the same willingness to be creative, as well as the ability to prioritize certain corporate cultural values over others. Complicating this process is the fact that many organizations, especially larger ones, are simply not equipped to provide the sort of creativity and flexibility patients need to perform their jobs. While money or prestige of title are indisputable incentives to join certain companies, chronically ill people sometimes need to readjust their criteria and choose an organization based on its culture instead. While a company's culture, priorities, and values are important to most workers, Rosalind Joffe feels chronically ill people need to factor them even more heavily than the average healthy employee would. In a way, this is another limiting factor for chronic workers since sometimes the best jobs for lucrative career advancement and the best jobs for health flexibility can't be found at the same place.

Brian's experience in the workplace is tangible proof that a company's attitude and values are an integral part of achieving workplace success as a chronically ill person. Not only did he initiate a dialogue about his cystic fibrosis from the outset, but that dialogue has continued to evolve over the several years he has worked at his company. For his part, Brian tries to schedule routine maintenance hospitalizations during slower times or around weekends as much as possible so his treatment doesn't disrupt the workflow. He also utilizes at-home IVs whenever he can so he can avoid going to the hospital altogether. Along with his proactive steps, his company has also responded in kind, allowing him to do certain parts of his job from home when his health keeps him out of the office.

"I'm really lucky, I know that. I'm working towards a position where I could pretty much always work remotely. It's a very conscious decision in terms of my health," he says, showing the same type of forward thinking Joffe helps her clients achieve. If it works out, Brian would be much better equipped to handle the disease progression he knows is in his future and still maintain his job.

As always, each individual patient's circumstances dictate the types of choices they can make and the type of choices they want to make. Sometimes the compromises we make to accommodate our health are especially painful, but knowing when and how to sacrifice professional gains for long-term health is something we can't afford to ignore.

23.

MEDICAL MAINTENANCE DOESN'T EQUAL HIGH MAINTENANCE

*Asking for accommodations may be
an art form, but it's also inevitable
for chronic consumers*

I USED TO BE THE TYPE OF PERSON who wouldn't send a dish back to the kitchen unless the chicken was blatantly pink or the steak still had a pulse. Fearful of being labeled difficult or demanding, I'd gingerly eat around the undercooked centers of meat or pick the avocado I'd mentioned I didn't want on my salad off the mountain of greens. Since I'm not at all shy about expressing my needs or desires in my own home, the fact that I often morphed into such a soft-spoken people-pleaser in public is somewhat perplexing to the people who know me best—in fact, I think my family would love it if I were that obsequious with them now and then.

So why did I act this way in service-related settings? I think it relates to the "good patient" complex I've discussed earlier. If I did stir up the gumption now and again to protest, it was accompanied by excessive apologies: "I'm so sorry to bother you. The chicken is delicious, but it's a bit too pink. I'm really sorry, I know it's a pain, but could I get it cooked a little more? I'm really sorry . . ."

And then I was diagnosed with celiac disease, and making special requests and asking a lot of questions at restaurants were no longer simply a matter of preference but of health. I'd grown up seeing my father bring his diet tonic water to restaurants, explaining he was diabetic and couldn't have regular tonic water, and I'd sat through countless meals where he negotiated sweet sauces to be placed on the side and starches to be replaced with green vegetables. He was always politely firm about his needs, and while I'd always marveled at that ability of his, I couldn't replicate it, whether my requests were based on personal preference or medical reasons—and I hadn't yet realized that both reasons were equally valid.

I'd always been somewhat of a healthy eater. I avoided anything fried, ate only low-fat dairy products, and cut down on starchy foods like pasta or bread in favor of whole grains. I was still an adventurous eater, though. I'd gone from the Italian and American cuisine of my childhood to dining out on sushi, spicy Thai soups, or monkfish wrapped in spinach and bacon by the time I was in my midtwenties.

After my diagnosis, I suddenly had to think about more than just the fat or sodium content in my food. I had to consider each individual ingredient, how it was prepared, and what possible contaminants it was cooked near. I didn't know what to ask, so I certainly couldn't expect restaurant staff to know how to answer me. The first few weeks of going gluten-free (GF), I opted out of these considerations altogether and simply ordered salad. When I was at home, I reached for the bagged lettuce and red onion, and I avoided buying much else at the grocery store. I had salad everywhere I went, every meal I ate, until no amount of dressing or freshly ground pepper could hide the fact that I was so sick of greens I'd rather go hungry than order another one.

If I ever wanted to enjoy a meal that didn't revolve around lettuce and balsamic vinegar, I needed to take action. I bought cookbooks and GF manuals and became familiar with the list of unsafe food items. I figured out how to buy groceries at Whole Foods without breaking the bank (avoid the pricey but delicious hot-food bar and look for the store brand). I experimented with new recipes and online GF stores, and most important, I learned from my mistakes: The first time I ate sushi after going gluten-free, I couldn't figure out why I got so sick afterward. You can't go wrong with raw fish and rice, right? Then I remembered the soy sauce, which most definitely contains wheat flour, and never made that mistake again. Whenever I eat sushi, I come armed with a little container of gluten-free soy sauce—just like my father with his plastic bottles of diet tonic water.

More than that, I began to see why it didn't embarrass my father to cater to his health needs and patrol the amount of sugar in his meals. If I didn't speak up and wound up ingesting gluten after all my hard work at removing it from my system, I'd be the one suffering later, not the waiter, the chef, or anyone else who could potentially be put out by my questions and accommodations. The fact that I was the one with the vested interest here supplanted all previous hesitation at being perceived as "difficult" or demanding. Like my father, I was politely firm, emphasis on politely, and I realized that asking for accommodations doesn't make you difficult—the tone and attitude with which you request them does.

Since going out to eat was a staple of my relationship with my then boyfriend and now husband, John, it was important to me to make it a successful experience. The more prepared and knowledgeable I was, the easier it was to translate my needs. When possible, I checked out menus online beforehand, making a short list of items I thought were "safe," and if that list was too short, I moved on to a new restaurant and a new menu. Sometimes I even called ahead to make sure accommodations could be made for me. I learned to be specific about what I couldn't have. Since not everyone knows what gluten is or what items contain it, I made sure to say I couldn't have anything with wheat, flour, or barley—the items most likely to appear in a typical dinner entrée. When met with an apathetic "I don't think it has any flour," I would respond with an upbeat, "Well, do you mind confirming that for me? Thanks so much!"

Getting diagnosed with celiac disease gave me the gumption to be the educated, selective consumer I had every right to be all along. Proof that I have evolved from the shrinking violet who poked at disgusting pink chicken into someone far savvier? I'm more attuned to the special needs of others too. Now when I go to a restaurant with my parents, I am the first one to ask for a booth, since my mother can't sit in hard chairs with her back and shoulder problems, and I encourage her to bring her pillow into the restaurant with her.

Whether it's requesting substitutions because of food allergies, needing a glass of juice right away to ease a diabetic low, or requiring special chairs or seating arrangements to decrease unnecessary joint pain, chronic consumers are always going to have to negotiate accommodations. Most of the time the general public is willing to meet our specifications and respect our requests—but of course, we first have to respect those needs ourselves.

24.

MULTIPLE ILLNESSES, MULTIPLE SIGNALS

*In a busy world, learn to prioritize—
not ignore—the minor aches and the
major pains*

BETWEEN THE THREE OF US and our collective diseases, my parents and I are certainly doing our part to keep the pharmaceutical and health care industries churning along. And we're not alone in our multiple-disease reality— over 125 million Americans are estimated to have a chronic illness, and more than half this number have more than one condition.[1] The millions of you out there juggling multiple conditions know how difficult it can be to manage all those symptoms, treatments, and complications at once and still hold down jobs and nurture relationships. In fact, it's nearly impossible, and inevitably some symptoms are ignored or discounted, even if they shouldn't be.

This challenge of managing too much information is very closely paralleled in the society in which we live. For chronic patients, the bombardment of facts and information to consider is as ever-present as the ticker tape on CNN or the "ping!" announcing yet another new e-mail in our in-box. On any given day, my body can send me the following messages in the form of symptoms: cough, wheeze, tightness in the chest, fatigue, clamminess, joint pain, tissue pain, stiffness, etc. Sometimes, I'll pick up only a couple of these messages, and sometimes they all shout at me at once—either way, I still need to decide which one deserves the most attention.

Jenni faces the same challenge. Managing the chronic pain and fatigue of fibromyalgia in addition to asthma and Raynaud's phenomenon translates into a sensory overload that she needs to sort through on a daily basis, focusing on the most significant or routine-altering symptoms and shelving the lesser concerns for another time. Usually, this is a great system; who is better attuned to the needs and demands of our bodies on a daily (even hourly) basis than we are? I know that my respiratory conditions and their complications will take precedence over the rest of my problems most of the time. My muscle pain may be more intense some days, for example, but when it comes to dealing with chronic pain or acute respiratory struggles, there's no choice: pain I can live with, oxygen I cannot live without.

I see the same tendencies in my parents. My mother forgot to tell me for a couple of months that an MRI had shown spots on her liver, not because she's careless or reckless, but because she was too consumed with her immediate health concerns—severe nerve pain from back problems—to focus on it. Sometimes my father takes a bit longer than his scheduled six weeks to get another IV infusion of medication for his connective tissue disease, not because he is nonchalant about sticking with his treatment, but because sometimes all the appointments he needs to make for his cardiac problems and diabetes take up time normally allotted for polymyositis. These examples are emblematic of the constant juggling routine that constitutes living with multiple illnesses: as soon as one flare subsides or one infection dissipates, something else emerges.

The problem is, the longer you've been ill and the more conflicting conditions you have to assemble into some sort of hierarchy, the more likely it becomes that you're a little *too* adept at filtering out physical complaints that might deserve attention now and again. Just because something isn't life-threatening or hugely incapacitating doesn't mean you should ignore it. As someone who once backpacked through Europe with torn ligaments in my ankle and competed in a skating tournament with a strep infection that had spread to my knee, I know this is much easier said than done.

The best way to correct this overcompensation? Compare your reaction to a healthy person's perspective on the same issue. I know you're thinking, "But a healthy person doesn't have twenty different things wrong! A healthy person would think something small is a really big deal!" I hear you. But sometimes, the healthy can serve as unwitting litmus tests, and isn't that what we need? Not just something to help plod through all the facts and information, but something (or someone) to help evaluate them?

Not wanting to deal with the rigmarole that accompanies any type of diagnostic endeavor, Jenni dismissed the frequent bruises that had sprouted all over her body for months for seemingly no reason. At the time, she was in the midst of a severe chronic pain flare, and exhausted from that, she couldn't tackle yet another problem and didn't want to find out something else was wrong that would require attention and energy on her part. She finally yielded to her husband's suggestion that she mention the bruises to her physician. Once she made the decision to address the problem, she snapped into efficient patient mode, insisting her doctor take it seriously and order the appropriate blood tests. As she suspected, the cause wasn't serious—the Advil she'd been taking for her pain made her blood clot less efficiently, and all she needed to do was stop taking Advil.

"That cleared up the whole problem, but my hesitation meant I was bruised all summer, right in bathing suit season," Jenni recalls. "Some issues aren't as pressing, but they're still important," she says, highlighting the central conflict of multiple conditions. If even the less-pressing issues are important—which they are—then how do we respond to competing strands of urgency?

A recent trip to the podiatrist's office to get new orthotics made me realize how imperative this counterbalance is. Once inside the exam room, the doctor and I spent the requisite amount of time going over my medical history, starting first with the chronic conditions, then the joint problems. Everything was going fine with the physical exam until he put pressure on my left heel. I yelped. He put pressure on my right heel. This time I winced.

"So you have heel pain? When does it bother you?" he asked.

I said it hurt every morning when I woke up and put my feet on the ground for the first time and any time I walked without wearing my orthotics and sneakers. It had been like that for a couple of years. I hadn't realized just how annoying a problem my heels had become or how much my heel pain affected my normal, daily routine until someone with a completely different perspective pointed it out to me.

My doctor ultimately diagnosed me with plantar fasciitis, a condition where the tissue connecting the heel bone to the toes is inflamed and tight. Left untreated, it can lead to more-complicated problems like heel spurs or the rupture of the Achilles tendon. It is not major, but it is something worth recognizing. I have enough to worry about; something as simple as being able to walk from the bedroom to the bathroom without limping in pain doesn't need to be on the list.

25.

SICK CHIC

*Being sick and being stylish are not
mutually exclusive*

IT WAS A FRIDAY NIGHT IN BOSTON, finally far enough into spring that we could shed our scarves and wool coats but still brisk enough that we couldn't break out our strappy sandals or sleeveless shirts just yet. My friends and I were gathered in a surprisingly upscale bar just outside Fenway Park, where gritty baseball fans and overdressed yuppies vied for tables and drank sugar-rimmed martinis and beers. It was the end of April and we were there to celebrate my birthday and catch up; with most of us in grad school or working full time, we could go weeks without seeing each other. It was a night to act—and more important, look—like a healthy person.

"You look really cute, so put-together," my friend Nicole said to me earlier that night as I got into her car. I was wearing a bright turquoise shell, brown cardigan, and brown corduroy skirt. I wore turquoise and other blue jewelry and had a patterned scarf in my hair to accent the color splash. I hadn't felt well enough to do much more than go to school and work and come home again in over a month, so I figured I should attempt to make an effort. Normally, I changed into sweatpants and a T-shirt as soon as I walked through my front door, so putting on "going out" clothes was an event. This outfit was the ultimate compromise in function versus form; it looked put-together but felt easy.

I thanked Nicole for her compliment, knowing that as a longtime friend and a health professional, she understood what it took for me to get dressed up and go out when I had no energy. I appreciated her subtlety in acknowledging that. Little did she know how strategic my outfit was, however. I'd planned the whole ensemble around wearing my low-heeled leather boots, which automatically meant I couldn't wear jeans or pants—I'm so short I need a higher heel to keep my hem from dragging on the ground.

"Don't tell anyone, but these are Easy Spirits," I said somewhat sheepishly, pointing down to my boots. "I couldn't deal with uncomfortable heels."

"Please, who cares if they're Easy Spirits? I'd never have known," she said, the same response another friend gave me when I handed her the same admission later that evening.

I looked around at the group of my friends and saw little difference between their healthy countenances and my own. Perhaps I'd finally pulled off accommodating my body without sacrificing all semblance of style?

Between sore quad muscles, a reconstructed right ankle, tendonitis-ridden hips, and the plantar fasciitis in my heels, I'd never been the best candidate for the spindly shoes most of my friends wear. Invariably, by the time I made it to the subway stop around the corner in heels, I was already uncomfortable, and within an hour of leaving my house, I was hobbling around in pain. It got to the point where my husband groaned when he saw me furrowing through my closet in search of a particular pair of heels, knowing a long, slow night was ahead of him if he couldn't talk me out of wearing them. I spent more time looking for my wedding shoes—twenty-seven pairs in four stores—than I spent looking for the dress itself. Even still, the wedding shoes were somewhat of a debacle; I was limping so terribly by the time the reception started that the catering manager slipped me a pair of chunky butterscotch pumps that miraculously happened to fit me and were covered by the hem of my wedding gown so no one was the wiser.

I'd made the pragmatic decision to buy comfortable footwear after the wedding shoe incident, but I hadn't committed to the Easy Spirits emotionally yet. Sure I read magazines and knew labels and cared about looking marginally presentable, but I was fairly low-maintenance—I'd rather buy books than get manicures, I do my grocery shopping in sweatpants and sneakers, and I had no clue about diamond carats until after my future husband, John, placed a sparkly ring complete with a family heirloom diamond on my finger. For me, my reluctant admission that I'd crossed over to the dark side of "sensible shoes" had less to do with fashion than it did with the fact that I often felt so run-down and didn't want my appearance to match my physical state. Gimpy joints aside, my constant wheezing and congestion and accompanying fatigue made me feel old and dilapidated—I once joked that I felt like a crumbling, peeling Victorian on a block of brand-new stainless steel and granite neo-Colonials. Internally, I felt frumpy in my broken-down body and out of touch with my peers, and I was loath to do anything to magnify those feelings outwardly.

However, I had to admit I was a lot more confident when I wasn't hobbling around crouched in pain. It was hard enough to commit to plans and actually follow through with them; why make the process more complicated? If style is some sort of indicator of personality or values, then at least mine reflected self-awareness, and finally, balance. I still have my rows of shiny, strappy heels, but I've added a lot more shoes that I can wear without grimacing as well. True, my conversion coincided with a sudden proliferation of ballet flats and kitten heels in magazines and in stores, but I chalked that up to serendipity. It's not about sacrificing personality or giving in; it's about making even the smaller decisions that are in our best interest.

26.
THE MAINTENANCE MODE
MYTH

Crises are difficult, but so is adjusting
to "normal" life without them

LIKE MANY OF YOU, a lifetime of illness left me all too familiar with medical emergencies and the upheaval that followed them. In fact, by the time I reached my early twenties, that was the only way of living I had known. In the ensuing calm, I began to realize just how well I'd always worked in crisis mode. During life-threatening moments, I knew what to do and how to stay nonplussed. As a college student, I studied for finals and wrote newspaper articles from the ICU. In graduate school, I taught writing classes so fresh from being discharged that I still had a hospital bracelet on my arm. And all of this seemed perfectly reasonable to me. Why shouldn't it?

Soon it became clear that instead of the cycle of crisis followed by recovery followed by crisis that I'd always known, I was in a new place altogether, something I have dubbed "maintenance mode." No longer would I have to exist in a state of precariousness punctuated by fleeting moments of predictability—I could actually join the ranks of "normal" people who went to work and went out when they pleased. I could make tentative plans for holidays or special occasions and believe that I really might be able to follow through; I could commit to freelance projects and anticipate completing them. I noticed that I stopped throwing in the caveats "unless I'm in the hospital" or "unless I get too sick" whenever plans were discussed, proof to me that I no longer felt I was merely waiting for the next disaster to unfold.

But don't let the obvious benefits of maintenance mode lull you into thinking that transitioning into it is either natural or easy. In many ways, the transition is really difficult— something I hadn't expected. I had no practical experience in setting limits for myself. Making up huge amounts of schoolwork on my own or staying up until dawn to catch up on work were basically the only ways I knew how to succeed. I'd never had a complete semester or uninterrupted stint at a job, and however grateful I was for my newfound stability, I really had no clue how to function within it: I didn't know what was a reasonable amount of time to spend grading essays since I'd never had the chance to budget my time of my own accord. I wasn't sure how much time I should allocate to my writing because I usually only got to it in spurts, that precious time in between infections. I wondered if I was crazy for agreeing to teach an additional writing course. I hadn't realized how much of my personality was wrapped up in the extremes of bedridden or overdrive that had carried me well into my twenties. Intensity followed me into recovery mode, where I scraped and scratched to catch up to where my life had left off while I had the chance. Suddenly, I had all this intensity bottled up and I wasn't sure where I was supposed to channel it anymore.

Apparently, I am not naturally wired for "calm," but I wonder if that's true for a lot of chronically ill people. I know I see the same pattern of crisis and recovery in my parents— my father is either working sixty-hour weeks or is laid up in bed because he's experiencing a polymyositis flare and can't move his muscles, and my mother is either running around doing errands and volunteering for the church or she is curled up on the couch, unable to uncoil her stiff, wrenched joints. In some ways, this relieves me because I am clearly not the only one maniacally compelled to live in extremes, but it also chastens me because I realize that since chronic illness is never going to disappear, this ugly pattern I know all too well will always lurk in the background.

When I first went into maintenance mode, everyone around me was encouraged and comforted by the realities of what was happening: "It's been two months since you've been in the hospital," they'd say, or "Wow, you made it to Thanksgiving *and* Christmas this year!" Of course I shared in their enthusiasm. But what I couldn't articulate to anyone was the sense that I didn't totally recognize myself anymore. I'd had twenty years to define myself within the parameters of crisis and recovery; a few months of relative calm wasn't enough time to recast my entire approach toward living, and it was unreasonable of me to expect that of myself.

On a deeper level, there were other maintenance mode myths that proved challenging. I'd never had the downtime to evaluate how my baseline health status had changed over the years. It was great to spend much less time in hospitals, yet it was almost as tough to see for the first time what "everyday" health meant for me: lots of wheezing, trouble breathing, fatigue. I stopped looking at life in terms of "getting back to normal" and realized that this new reality *was* my normal. I also realized how dangerous my former definition of "crisis" was. If I wasn't two seconds away from intubation, then it wasn't serious.

It's now been about two years since I first tasted stability, and I am pleased to report I am much more comfortable with it. Obviously, maintenance mode will never be permanent, but if we're lucky enough to achieve it now and then, we can learn a lot from it.

27.

TO ACCEPT OR DENY

*Acceptance isn't easy but it signals
wisdom, not defeat*

T HE PHRASE "ACCEPTING LIMITATIONS" has always irrationally annoyed me, got right under my skin
the way pencil-thin capri pants, toy poodles, and tapered
jeans with white sneakers always did. In my head, it
conjured up visions of saccharine self-help manuals and
smiling elderly women with knitting needles on their laps using Stannah stairlifts to get upstairs in commercials. Those
images had nothing to do with me. I didn't want to be serene
and yielding, and I'd run myself ragged over the years, often
at the expense of my health, to prove this.

But what happens when the physical symptoms finally
outweigh our determination to ignore them? There's a huge
difference between simply acknowledging limitations caused
by health conditions and actually responding to them in a
productive way. Denial was my preferred default method for
years, and while I think a certain amount of denial is

necessary to get by, the process of acceptance really depends on moderation and maturation.

Acceptance means something different to each patient and each particular manifestation of illness. For Kerri and the millions of people who have diabetes, the daily reminders of the condition are one obstacle. The highs and lows of blood sugar and the testing and planning are always there, as is the fluctuation between the immediate gratification of eating something sweet and starchy and the implicit awareness that the choices you make in the present have long-term consequences. If you get too bogged down in worrying about the future, it's difficult to enjoy the present; yet if you're too casual about managing the disease now, your health will be that much more affected later in life.

This same conundrum can be applied to most chronic illnesses, certainly, but Kerri distinguishes another aspect of acceptance in relation to diabetes: the fine line between sustaining necessary hope for a cure and not hoping so much that you neglect the requirements of the disease in the present. For her, a cure was always something that would happen in the future: in grade school, it was something that would happen during high school—she joked that it would be like getting a diploma and a pancreas—and in high school, it would happen in college, and so on.

"You don't lose hope for a cure so much as the expectation of a cure," she explains, likening the idea of a cure to the carrot that dangles proverbially in front of her. It's tantalizing, but it can't supplant the everyday mechanics of living with diabetes. To view her disease through the benchmark of a cure would fail to account for the many successes in her life professionally and personally, as well as the daily victories over the challenges of diabetes.

If accepting certain realities about chronic diseases like diabetes requires nuanced shifts in attitude or expectation, then what does the process look like for people with serious illnesses that, in the end, are neither curable *nor* treatable? Brian was just ten years old when his doctor explained to him the difference between "chronic" and "terminal," and his understanding of his ultimately terminal illness has shaped much of the way he has lived his life.

"As soon as you realize you have a time limit on your life, you start thinking about things differently than kids your age—you grow up fast. But then it goes full circle; there comes a point where you know it's going to happen, but what are you going to do about it?" he says.

A perennial partier—"if you're not living, you're dying" is emblematic of his attitude toward life—he still makes sure he goes out every chance he gets and never turns down an opportunity to have fun. But now that he's older and his disease has progressed, he is a lot more diligent about taking care of himself. It's a constant battle between denial and pragmatism; nothing makes him *feel* like he is sick more than using his nebulizer or having chest PT, yet to avoid those things would only make him feel worse. As much as he'd like to, he cannot afford to ignore the very real manifestations of illness in his life.

However, the crux of Brian's evolution into being a more conscientious patient and his acceptance of the physical trappings of illness is not something that can be explained away by disease progression alone. So what else has changed? He has also realized how much his health impacts the people around him, from his family to his friends to the people he has dated, a realization that is a lot easier to make at twenty-five than when he was in grade school, college, or even just starting out in the professional world. "It would be sort of selfish of me not to take care of myself," he says, and in his case, taking care of himself means paying attention to all the things his disease management requires, regardless of whether it reminds him yet again that he has a terminal illness. Generally, the older you get, the more awareness you have of other people's needs and the more entrenched in relationships you become. For people like Brian who have grown up with serious illness, such a shift in perspective is bound to occur as emotional, intellectual, and social needs and awareness develop.

It's not a question of accepting CF in his life. Most of his decisions, from his job status to his friends to his hectic social life, have always been made precisely with CF in mind. "CF is as much a part of me as any of my other characteristics. It's pretty definitive of who I am," Brian says. Acceptance, then, doesn't constitute living in the shadow of eventual death, nor does it entail blithely dismissing the realities of his condition. Acceptance means integrating the tedious daily rigors of illness not simply because you are supposed to, but also because you recognize there is more at stake in your wellness than your own feelings.

In my case, I pinpoint exactly when I shifted from being someone who took on too much, and ignored even more just to prove I could, to being someone who was more realistic and mature about my options. By my second year of graduate school, my health was the main determinant in virtually every decision I made, from larger issues like did I have the stamina for a nine-to-five career and if I could (or should) have children to the mundane decision of whether I should bring the L. L. Bean backpack or the leather shoulder bag to school with me in the morning—the latter was much more professional, but the former balanced the weight of my books and files and made it easier to breathe.

One October day of that year, my then-fiancé, John, lugged all my grocery bags up my street since I couldn't carry any of them. The sheer ludicrousness of not carrying my own bags got to me. How long had it been since I'd had the lung capacity to carry my groceries? I couldn't even remember. Or since I'd gone clothes shopping and been able to get my purchases home on foot? Or since I'd been able to load suitcases in my car or move boxes? Add the muscle weakness and fatigue from my recent adrenal failure, and I felt pretty much useless.

"When did it get to the point where I have to *think* to breathe?" I asked him, slamming the apartment door shut behind me and throwing my keys onto the coffee table. The simplicity—and accuracy—of the question shocked both of us.

He didn't answer, and held me in his arms instead. As he hugged me, I wondered what else I'd chosen not to notice. I knew that all those years of infections, respiratory distress, collapsed lungs, and suffocating phlegm were not caused by asthma. Combined with my other medical problems, the diagnosis of PCD took all those mishmashed symptoms and loose ends and packaged them in a way that made total sense. But did I really think acronyms like PCD were just labels, that knowing what was going on with my body was merely a cerebral act? Knowing is supremely emotional too.

I hadn't responded to the physical progression of my diseases by changing my mental approach at all. I was still repeating the same mistakes from college and even from high school. I took on too many jobs and got so run down that my infections and other conditions were exacerbated further. I would then have to quit something, which would frustrate me so much that I'd soon find another commitment to take on just to show that I could. Mature, yes?

Obviously my body couldn't take this anymore, but that wasn't the only thing that finally snapped me out of my old cycle. All the deliberations that guided my decisions were increasingly part of John's life too, a thought that weighed on me constantly. Packing carry-on luggage to visit his parents in Michigan for a weekend was an elaborate process of squeezing wallets and books in among all my medications, which filled up my backpack on their own. We had to streamline our clothes in our suitcase so we could pack my nebulizer in case I had trouble breathing. John lugged the heavy, bulky Vest—a stand-in for the times when I can't see my chest physical therapist, the Vest is basically a generator with two tubes that connects to a vest I buckle myself into that inflates with air and "shakes" me to loosen the mucus in my lungs—through airport terminals and bus stations.

There were more than logistical implications for John. His quality of life and happiness were increasingly connected to mine. The sicker I was, the worse it was for him too, and it wasn't fair of me to ignore the aspects of my illnesses that I could control. Being realistic about my limitations did not equal being negative or weak, I slowly discovered; it meant being fair to my body and fair to the people who cared about me. In a way, such an awareness is the natural next step in the growing evolution of the chronically ill young adult—the responsibilities, obligations, and challenges that characterized surviving academia and the workplace follow each and every one of us home. Acceptance is the intersection where the consequences of our public identities collide with our personal ones.

A few weeks after that October day, I cut back on my teaching schedule for the coming semester and chose not to take on additional courses that summer so I would be in more optimal health for our upcoming wedding. I found that I didn't resent these choices the way I used to, because I felt in control of them and saw that their benefits for John and me far outweighed this ill-fitting logic that accepting limitations meant resignation. It meant making my own investment in our future, something that all of us living with chronic diseases must come to terms with in our own way.

PART 3

Personal Life: Illness and Relationships

Part Two

Detectives, Thieves, and Other Oddballs

28.

THE CHRONIC KID IS ALL GROWN UP

*You're no longer a sick kid, but don't
expect your parents to always see that*

IF APPRECIATING THE IMPACT OF ILLNESSES on the
people closest to us is the fundamental hallmark of an
adult perspective on illness, then it stands to reason that the
first place to explore this impact is the nuclear family, the
parents and siblings who've seen us through each stage of
sickness. For those of us who were chronically ill children,
our parents may have trouble no longer seeing us as sick
kids because we will always be their children and we will
always be sick. In ways both physical and emotional, our
parents were heavily involved and invested in our disease
management, and that investment doesn't end simply when
we get our drivers' licenses, come of legal age, go to college,
or enter into serious romantic commitments. Complicating
these boundaries is the fact that the relationship between
parents and chronically ill children is often especially close;

as Kerri puts it, when someone stands at the edge of your mortality and faces it with you as our parents have, it establishes a deep bond.

So what happens to that bond when we're adults who are fully capable of managing our conditions and making our own decisions?

Before I found my current specialist, the physician I saw postcollege was actually a pediatric pulmonologist. I was a "new patient" in peds at the age of twenty-three. Saddled with a bag of books and scattered notes, a cell phone, and a heavy dose of cynicism, I was an anomaly in the waiting room of rambunctious toddlers and their parents. As I sat there flipping through back issues of *Parent* magazine and dodging projectile blocks, a knot slowly coiled in my stomach. The toys, the artwork, the distractions the parents tried to provide—they were all too familiar for me. After I got my license and then moved away for college, neither of my parents had accompanied me to the doctor. Though I'd never admit it to her, being in a pediatric waiting room again made me wish my mother was there with me too. I saw clearly for the first time what all those years must have been like for my mother—how from the moment I was born and whisked away into the neonatal intensive care unit so much of her control and authority as a parent was also taken away, and how terrifying that must have been. She could do many things for me except for the one desire that consumed her most: to make me well.

Likewise, from Kerri's perspective as a twenty-eight-year-old, she can now imagine how scary it must have been for her mother to look at her formerly healthy six-year-old and wonder if she'd make it into adulthood and how her own choices and capabilities would influence her daughter's health. If she didn't provide Kerri with the right foods, would that mean her daughter would experience more eye and renal damage as an adult? If she didn't help Kerri educate her classmates and teachers about diabetes effectively, would her daughter's self-esteem suffer?

Our parents responded to our illness with action, a common (and in most cases, inevitable) reaction. Research suggests that the most effective coping strategies utilized by parents depend heavily on the nature of disease itself. Diseases like diabetes or respiratory illnesses, which require constant monitoring, necessitate different degrees of time, energy, and investment than chronic conditions characterized by more pronounced flares and corresponding asymptomatic periods.[1] It makes sense, then, that the more present a disease is in a family's life, the more defined all parties involved are by that disease. For my mother, action in response to these realities meant taking me to endless specialists and referrals, demanding certain medicines postsurgery to reduce my nausea, making sure my nebulizer was with me when I went on sleepovers, slipping into my room at night to see if my ears were draining blood and if I was breathing. Our relationship was less strictly parent-child than coconspirators, with illness serving as our common foe. When I was a child and needed someone to drive me to blood tests, take me to the emergency room, or hold me when I cried, this arrangement suited me well.

Logistically, mother had the time and flexibility to be the constant caregiver when I was young, but my father shouldered his own strain. He cried in private, in hospital corridors, thinking I couldn't hear him, in his car before he pulled out of the parking garage to go home from the hospital without me, thinking I wouldn't know. In public, he was boisterous, the first one to inquire why the wait was so long in the emergency room, the first to ask a doctor what else he or she was planning to try, the first to demand they do something, anything, to help me breathe, as if his speaking loudly enough would improve the treatment I received. As a result of his own illnesses, he knew intimately the physical and emotional toll illness took on a patient, and he wanted something different for me.

To this day, I think he is still haunted by an episode from my stint in isolation as a five-year-old. After a couple of weeks in the hospital, I'd run out of viable veins in both arms for my IV line. My parents nicknamed the deep blue and purple bruises the blown veins left on my skin "blue-berries," but the cheerful moniker did little to assuage my morbid fear of anyone coming near me with yet another needle. The day my nurse decided it was time to start using the veins in my ankles for my IV coincided with one of my father's after-work visits. I was terrified and put up a mighty fight, thrashing, crying, and squirming. When I attempted to kick the nurse in the face so she couldn't stick the needle in my foot, she turned to my father for help holding me down. With tears streaming down my face, I looked up at him and shrieked, "Why are you doing this? Don't you love me anymore?"

Being asked to do something that causes a child both physical and emotional pain because it is what's needed to help that child get well is the ultimate embodiment of what it means to be the parent of a sick child. In numerous and less dramatic ways, it was something my parents were asked to do over and over when I was a child, and I know it still compounds the guilt they already feel over the fact that my diseases are inherited.

Kerri says her mother became the "go-to girl" for all things diabetes-related. Learning how to plunge a syringe into Kerri's veins and mastering the many details and intricacies of managing type 1 diabetes fell to her parents, especially her mother. From introducing a diabetic diet for the household to sending Kerri to a diabetes camp where she could interact with other patients her own age, her mother made sure the immediate goals of diabetes management were met so that the long-term complications would be as minimal as possible. Since her mother was so immersed in management of the disease, in a sense it became their disease. Phrases like "We need to test our sugar" or "We need to take a nice long walk" were common when Kerri was growing up, and it wasn't until Kerri was a teenager and began to take more ownership over her care that she began to chafe at them. Looking back, she is wholly appreciative of all the things her parents did to keep her healthy and grounded, but sees the eventual transfer from "we" to "*I* need to do this to make sure I'm okay" as essential for any self-managed disease like diabetes. She now teases her mother about the "we" phenomenon, a joke she knows she can make without hurting her mother, because after all these years, her mother realizes Kerri is just as proactive and committed to managing her diabetes as she was when she was in charge of Kerri's health.

Looking back, I am amazed at the sheer amount of time my health needs consumed. If we weren't in a waiting room or shuttling to another surgery or test, I was home sick on the couch and my mother would shuffle around her carpooling duties for my hockey-playing older brothers or her commitments as a Hospice volunteer and the pastoral associate at our church. Either way, how I was feeling largely dictated both how she would feel and what she could do. As a child, I could really only focus on how these things affected me—it was *my* recital I missed, *my* friend's party I couldn't go to, *my* Christmas Eve that was marred by surgery—but now that I am an adult, I realize how strongly all these losses and sacrifices defined my parents as well.

"You have to understand, I've spent every waking moment of your life worrying about your health. Just because you're an adult doesn't mean I can just shut that off," my mother recently said to me. I was exasperated with her for telling me for the fifth time in two minutes to call my doctor and ask for a new medication when I'd already e-mailed him and taken care of the situation. It reminded me of when I was a kid and she would ask: "Did you take your medicine?" "Do you need your nebulizer?" and more frequently, "Are you sure you don't need to use the Vest again?" I told her that I was a twenty-six-year-old married woman and I'd managed myself, my medications, and my doctors' appointments for years. I *knew* what to do, and I knew my body better than anyone else.

With some distance from my immediate irritation, my mother's words forced me to consider how, for so many years, my illnesses had been just as much theirs. Since I was a teenager, I'd worked so hard to establish boundaries. I kept them updated on my doctors' appointments, I let them know about changes to my treatment plan, I filled them in on my latest insurance battle over coverage for chest PT, but only as secondhand participants. It didn't occur to me how hard that might have been for them.

At the same time, however annoyed I got in situations like that, I also realized that my parents understood what I'd been through and what my life was like better than anyone else possibly could. Like Kerri said, we'd faced mortality—in our case, both mine and my father's—together, and that connected us for life. When I was angry or frustrated or just sick of illness, they were the ones I called because I knew they had felt that way too. Despite how many years had passed, in many ways we were still coconspirators facing down a common enemy, and that struggle typifies the complexity of forging an adult relationship with your parents when there is a history of illness.

I actually found myself repeating my mother's words to my husband recently when we were discussing my parents' reaction to a recent bout of infections I'd had. They called constantly, asking all the usual questions about nebulizers and chest PT and the ever-present "How do you feel today?"

"Don't you think they're a little too involved, a little too close?" he asked. "Maybe they're making a bigger deal out of this than what's necessary?"

It was a conversation we had often as we navigated our newfound status as a married unit. My response was usually to agree with him while simultaneously acknowledging that their concern was well-intentioned. This time, though, I looked at the situation a bit differently.

"Since I was born, my illnesses have consumed their lives," I said. "Just because I can handle it on my own doesn't mean the worry magically disappears. They're used to being my support system and they don't have a channel for their worry anymore."

It occurred to me later that perhaps this was what it was like to truly be an adult—as a child, my needs and my illnesses came first and subsumed theirs. Now it was time for me to start putting their needs before mine in certain situations and recognize that my need to be independent doesn't always have to trump their need to be parents.

29.

THE RESPONSIBILITY TRAP

*Don't ignore the lifelong impact of
chronic illness on sibling dynamics*

Y OU KNOW, if anything ever happens and you need
help, I'll take care of you, right? If you're sick and in
trouble, you'll never be alone. I've told Mom and Dad that
so they don't worry about you and now I'm telling you,"
my older brother Michael told me over the phone one night.
It was during my first year of graduate school, and I'd recently been released from the hospital. The remark was
characteristic of Michael: completely sincere and completely
surprising—even though it shouldn't have been, because
that is how Michael works. He's cerebral and analytical, but
when he does say something emotional, however matter-of-
fact his delivery, you know there's a lot of thought and care
behind his words.

His remark was also indicative of the healthy sibling–sick
sibling dynamic. My two brothers have been my as-needed
caregivers, errand runners, and pinch-hitting hospital visitors

my entire life. There's an ever-increasing body of literature that explores the impact of chronic illness on the siblings of sick children, but what happens when we're all adults, busy with our own jobs, mortgage payments, and expanding families? A meta-analysis of data published in the *Journal of Pediatric Psychology* found that negative psychological functioning, like depression and anxiety, is found in siblings of chronically ill patients, who as children often have to take on caregiver roles and adapt to decreased parental attention and frequent disruptions in their daily lives.[1] The negative effect of this decreased parental attention obviously wanes as we age, but many of the same childhood responsibilities of healthy siblings remain the same into adulthood.

When Kerri was a child, diabetes bonded her and her parents together in a unique way that was not shared by her siblings. To her older brother and younger sister, diabetes was the reason the household diet changed, and the reason their mother hid ice-cream sandwiches in frozen vegetable bags and urged her nondiabetic children to have this special "broccoli" so they weren't totally deprived of fun food. They knew Kerri had to take insulin, they knew her parents worried about her in ways they didn't have to worry about them, but they didn't really understand what it meant to live with diabetes until Kerri was an adult and started her diabetes blog. "Now, they're both reading it and saying things like, 'I didn't *know*, I had no idea what it was really like,'" she says.

Perhaps this shift is the inevitable by-product of maturity; young children are naturally more self-involved and less likely to understand the fine points of someone else's health problems. Maybe it also speaks to Kerri's mother's ability to differentiate one daughter's disease from her healthy children's needs—if diabetes didn't infringe on their lives in hugely disruptive ways, then they didn't need to pay attention to it as much. Or perhaps as Kerri's own understanding of the role of diabetes in her life has evolved, her siblings' understanding has also grown in the same ways. Either way, her siblings' awareness of the diabetic experience has brought them closer now than living together as children did.

Marc and Michael are, respectively, five and eight years older than I am, and I know my illnesses had a more intrusive effect on their childhoods. One of my mother's most poignant stories from when we were little was when she first brought me home from the hospital. I was born prematurely and my lungs collapsed, so I was kept in an incubator for several weeks. When I was finally allowed to come home, Michael sensed, in his own little-boy way, that I was fragile. For days, he and his friend Johnny spent hours standing guard at my bassinette, moving only to switch sides with each other, as if to reassure my mother nothing would happen to me on their watch. When I was a little older, it was my brother Marc who gave me what I needed most at the time. He let me ride around the house on his back like a horse, he let me crimp his hair using a grooved curling iron, he even let me put nail polish on his nails one afternoon when I was bored and couldn't go outside to play because of an infection. I got a lot of attention from adults because I was always so sick, but rather than resenting it, my brothers gave me the kind of attention I subconsciously craved: they let me be a little sister, not just a sick little sister.

I also attribute their lack of resentment as children to the fact that my parents were diligent about making sure to spend one-on-one time with each brother, and that the boys had lots of outlets to form their own identities, things my illnesses couldn't touch—they played sports, had sleepovers and pizza parties, and always had a pickup game of street hockey going on with the neighborhood kids. I can only imagine how hard it was for my mother to work in Marc's and Michael's early-morning scrimmages, travel team schedules, and altar server classes at our church with all that she had to do for me when I was sick, but she did. Without so many outside activities and opportunities to feel good about their childhood, I think my brothers would have had a much harder time dealing with so much illness in their lives.

To my mother, a woman who has spent decades of her life bringing her loved ones to the hospital, the chapel has always been the most important place in the building. In a place where the gods of science reign supreme and what can be quantified counts, she seeks out the ineffable. She brought that same sense of spirituality home with her, and faith definitely molded our childhood dynamic as well.

Like my brothers, I am a product of a Catholic-school education from kindergarten through college (I have the plaid uniform and cautionary tales on the evils of cohabitation to prove it). When we were young, we went to church as a family every Sunday, we participated in youth choir and youth group activities, and no holiday was celebrated without appropriate deference to and respect for the religious aspects. My father's serious illnesses only strengthened my parents' already substantial faith, and that transferred onto us as well.

In our household, the knowledge that whatever challenges we were given were ones our God knew we could handle was sacrosanct. As children, we couldn't see things with that much enlightenment, but we knew my parents found solace through their faith and in our own age-appropriate ways, I think we found comfort too. Sure, my brothers complained about early-morning Mass and I pitched fits when I didn't like the dress my mother wanted me to wear to the service, but our church gave us a place to belong to, something for all of us to self-identify with that wasn't overshadowed by illness. In fact, faith made illness seem much less threatening.

Without any of us ever speaking about it directly until that night Mike vocalized it on the phone, I already knew I'd never be alone. Do I feel guilty that my brothers need to think in these terms, that illness has tethered me to them even now? Definitely, just like I feel guilty about all the times my parents had to focus on me, the nights and weeks in the hospital and the days I was home sick when they were with me instead of watching my brothers play sports or do things with them when we were children. It doesn't matter what the particular illness is; there's no way a sick kid doesn't drain parental time and energy at the expense of the healthier siblings. Our situation was compounded since I wasn't even the only patient. By the time I was a toddler, my brothers had already lived through my father's near-death experiences with cancer and polymyositis. I now realize that there was never a time where they *didn't* know illness, where it didn't somehow define what they could do and what they knew.

I remember the weeks I spent in isolation when I was five, and the familiar memories of the IV tubes, the view of the Charles River out of my window, my mother sitting in her blue leather chair every day. I recall my mother calling my aunt's house in Pennsylvania at night to check on my brothers, where they had been shipped until my mother and I could come home from the hospital. I remember being jealous they went to water parks and carnivals while I was stuck in a hospital bed, but now that I'm older, I can see the other side of the telephone line: two scared little boys who missed their parents and their friends, who missed sleeping in their own beds and who couldn't do that because their sister was sick. They may not have liked it, but they never treated me like they blamed me for it.

That same connection has evolved with us. As I grew older, they spent nights on the phone, counseling me through high school traumas, college fears, and long hospital stays. They flew down to stay with me when I was an inpatient in college, and still juggled holiday meals with their in-laws with visiting me in the hospital on Christmases and Thanksgivings and Easters when I couldn't be with them otherwise. They both have beautiful daughters of their own, and the first question I asked each of them when they came out of the delivery room was, "Is she healthy? How are her lungs?" *Please don't let her be like me.* I know my brothers have the skills and the knowledge to be superb caretakers if their children were sick, but I am so relieved they don't have to be—they've already put in too much time caring for sick relatives.

As much as I feel guilty for the time, attention, and relative normalcy I've taken from them over the years, I also feel incredibly fortunate to have siblings who "get it" as much as healthy people can, who understand the unpredictable nature of chronic illness, who recognize that in many ways, John's and my life is a lot more complicated than most people think. I wonder if this sense of relief is how Kerri felt when her adult siblings began to have a more comprehensive and realistic understanding of life with diabetes. My brothers have seen enough of the downside of chronic illness to appreciate that the bond illness has formed between my parents and me is something they can never be a part of, but they wouldn't have traded being healthy for being the center of our parents' anxious attention.

I hope I don't ever need to take Michael up on his offer. I hope the intrusions of my illnesses are limited to occasional hospital visits and phone calls. Like so many families with chronic illness, we already spent an entire childhood with health problems punctuating our existence, and I don't want that legacy to follow us through adulthood—but it's reassuring to know that the same protective buffer I had as a child is there if I ever need it again.

30.
THE CHRONIC COMIC

Humor can integrate—not
obfuscate—illness for our healthy
friends

WHEN I WAS GROWING UP, my illnesses made me a walking hodgepodge of injuries, ailments, and oddities. When I was at home, I knew that I was safe and that my brothers wouldn't tease me, but once I left our insular little world, I felt this difference acutely. I tried to prevent others from being the ones to call out my differences, usually by invoking humor and nonchalance.

Consider the summer between my fourth and fifth grades: I had a green and white air cast on my right ankle, the result of a severe sprain. Its bottom was ragged and torn from being dragged along the bare pavement, and granules of rock were permanently trapped in the gel inserts. My left wrist had fractured again, the bones as brittle as small twigs from the steroids I took to help my breathing. I chose hot pink for my arm cast this time, and autographs and smiley faces were plastered across it in thick, black permanent marker. I still had bruises up and down my "good" arm from unsuccessful blood draws, adding some more color to my mélange. I knew it was going to be a long summer unless I adopted my default strategy: crack jokes and sarcastic comments, pretend nothing is amiss, and whatever else happens, make them laugh with me before they feel awkward or laugh *at* me.

One morning, before heading to the beach, I settled my air cast almost all the way into my sparkly jelly shoes, stuck a magenta scrunchie in my ponytail to match my arm cast, and threw a garbage bag in my backpack to wrap around my arm in the water. I walked down the street leading to the beach with my childhood best friend, who was a good six inches taller and tanned and sinewy. As we passed all the people waiting in line for the ice-cream truck, I swallowed deeply, steeling myself for the inevitable comments. Just before we were parallel with the crowd, I developed a sort of swagger to my lopsided gait and ever so casually smirked and said loudly enough for the entire crowd to hear, "You shoulda seen the other guy."

I'd pilfered the line from a leathered old man smoking outside the post office the day before. He'd looked at me and removed the cigarette from his mouth, his smirk revealing several missing teeth. "Christ, sweetheart, what happened to you? And what's the other guy look like? I hope you got him good!" What can you say to that? Trying to look dignified in decidedly undignified circumstances, I stared straight in front of me and walked—limped, really—by him.

"It was ugly," I now added, nodding at my friend in that "you know what I'm talking about" kind of way. In my wake, I heard assorted chuckles.

It was working.

I have often wondered whether my particular approaches toward dealing with chronic illness tread a fine line between effective coping mechanism and denial. To me, they're mutually inclusive. My biggest concern has always been that I do not want my illness to define or overwhelm my relationships. As a child, I believed if we could all laugh about it, there was nothing to worry about, so humor was more about protecting me than anyone else. The more serious my illnesses became, the more difficult it was to keep these darker shadows from casting a pall over my relationships. I now see that not everything can always be couched in terms that are light and that to try to do so is a disservice to them and to our relationships.

Now I no longer rely solely on humor as a vehicle to avoid accepting the consequences of illness in my life. In the past, while I was cracking jokes and dismissing my illness, I was also frustrated that most of my friends did not understand how I was feeling. I was isolated by my own attempts to entertain them. I didn't fully realize how the internal world of illness intersects with the external world of relationships, and that's something that ultimately we all need to recognize. You can process the supremely individual parts of illness in private and still share what is necessary and accessible to others. Personally, the most effective way I know how to share that information is through humor, except that now the humor allows for honesty as well as denial.

I practice a delicate process of checks and balances, a system designed to make sure all needs are met—mine, those of my family, and those of my friends. I try to familiarize my problems to people by presenting them in terms that aren't scary, threatening, or heavy-handed. It is a constant redrawing of boundaries, a line that changes as frequently as my oxygen saturation and rate of infection. My friends and I refer to my nebulizer and oxygen face mask in the hospital as the "Super Bong," and to them, it is no longer intimidating. The fall after college graduation, when I didn't feel well enough to go out on weekends for three months, we referred to it as my Boo Radley phase, in honor of the hermetic recluse in *To Kill a Mockingbird*. My friends admire the variety of colors in the "track marks" left by IVs and ask if my medications require their own carry-on bag when I travel (they do).

They take their cues from me, and when I am able to make light of it, they know that they can too. They joke about putting me in an all-purpose bubble so I'll stop getting infections, and I joke about feeling guilty for being an organ donor because I'm not sure many of my organs would actually improve someone's health. Maybe my gallbladder is an option, I tell them, because so far nothing has happened to my gallbladder. Of course, the irony is that the gallbladder is a nonessential organ.

The more I've started to let my friends in by choice and by necessity, the more they have embraced my illness. There is no end to the things they have done for me in recent years: taking shifts sleeping beside my hospital bed in college, postponing work or other commitments to be with me, driving me to appointments, calling, visiting, bringing my favorites things (books, magazines, and chai lattes) to the hospital, celebrating with me when I feel well. Most aren't squeamish or embarrassed by the tubes, needles, or chest PT. In fact, some of them have even learned how to do chest PT for me in case of emergency. They have grown to see that some days I can barely walk, while others I will take charge of organizing our plans—like me, they are now conditioned to take it day by day, if not hour by hour. I am much more relaxed knowing there is no pressure on me to be healthy or even to be funny.

I've also learned to distinguish when I can be direct and when it is better to make some topics lighter for certain people. People who are in health care or are used to hospitals typically ask a lot of questions about the specifics of my health and are totally comfortable on an inpatient floor. When talking with people who are less familiar with my conditions or don't like hospitals, I usually use less detail and more humor to couch the unknown and make it less threatening. They are the ones who are more likely to say things like "Let me know if I can run any errands for you" rather than "So what does that mean in terms of your prognosis?" and they are willing, even happy, to do such favors. They are also the ones who need a smile or a laugh from me to know everything will be okay.

Knowing the adaptive styles of our friends and healthy counterparts is just as important as their understanding of our own. Selective humor is beneficial for some, but blanket humor is counterproductive for all.

31.

CHRONIC SOCIALITES

Illness doesn't have to mean isolation

O NE OF THE ONLY PREDICTABLE things about
chronic illness is its unpredictability, and one of the
most frustrating consequences of being sick is the impact of
that unpredictability on our social lives. It's difficult enough
to make plans that work for groups of people with busy
schedules, but throw in something like a fibromyalgia pain
flare, an exacerbation of gastrointestinal problems, a migraine, or extreme fatigue or inflammation, and suddenly
socializing gets that much more complicated. Addressing
illness demands and still maintaining friendships and social
activities is a process that requires creativity, flexibility, and
most important, trust in the very people you fear disap-
pointing.

I enjoy planning events and get-togethers; from small
dinner parties to drinks and appetizers out to large holiday
celebrations, it's always been important to me to get groups
of people together. I wonder how much this tendency is, like

so many other characteristics, in some ways a response to the presence of illness itself. Perhaps planning and organizing is a way of seeking control over the very circumstances that are so often out of my control. Either way, the greatest irony is that very often, I am the one who winds up not being able to make the events or plans I've initiated.

Such failed missions include the plays and shows I bought tickets for and never attended, the trips to Connecticut or New York City for friends' birthdays I opted out of at the last minute three years in a row, the baptism of my friend's first baby I had to leave early, the going-away party I missed because I had yet another infection. I'm sure many of you can relate to special-event remorse like this, but the more everyday letdowns can be equally frustrating. It is the Friday-night drinks and the Saturday group dinners in my own city that I often miss, and I absolutely dread dialing someone's phone number and starting the "I'm really sorry but . . ." speech. I feel bad enough when I don't make it to the big-ticket birthday getaways and the showers for other people—especially since they've done that for me—but I also feel foolish when I send out e-mails asking if people want to meet at a certain restaurant the following week and then I don't attend.

The older I've gotten, the more cancellations I've accumulated—an inevitable by-product of certain symptoms worsening and other more temporary conditions (like adrenal depletion) flaring. Illness progression is an obvious part of the scenario, but there's also something about the social milieu of young professionals and postcollege life that contributes to it. For one thing, plans are much more structured since everyone has busy schedules and multiple commitments; very rarely do I find myself hanging out with friends on the spur of the moment. For another, many people are married or in serious romantic relationships now. They're also juggling graduate school, building careers, and often traveling a lot more. Outings with so much negotiation and consideration behind them are that much more frustrating to have to miss.

In recent years, there have been stretches of time when I backed out of plans far more than I actually followed through with them. When I was twenty-four, I spent an entire semester's worth of weekends on my couch, too run down from adrenal failure and infections to do anything besides stare listlessly at the television. I stopped making plans altogether, thinking it was more annoying to constantly have to call my friends and cancel than it was to never have any plans in the first place.

One of the many problems with this attitude is that it failed to consider the definition of friendship—it's a two-sided relationship. Where was my friends' say in this unilateral decision to remove myself?

My friends have years of hospital visits, phone calls, and errands run behind them. Clearly, these were people who understood my situation, and people who were not deterred by illness. I was the one with the guilt complex, and indulging in it to the extent that I stopped making any plans at all wasn't fair to the people who had earned a lot more credit than that. I decided a more proactive approach to socializing was in order. I started inviting my friends to my house more often since that was easier than traveling to other locales if I didn't feel up to it. I also stopped being stubborn and began suggesting meeting at restaurants and bars that were either closer to my part of the city or had parking so that if I didn't feel well, I could at least cut down on my commute. I'd been hesitant to directly express certain preferences or accommodations before because I didn't want our plans to become "my" plans, but I began to see that the location wasn't nearly as important to everyone else as the simple act of seeing each other.

With over a decade of living with fibromyalgia behind her, Jenni has made huge strides in terms of finding that elusive balance between catering to her specific physical needs and remaining part of her circles of friends. There are always days when her pain is too pronounced to venture out of her house, but even then she still connects with them by phone, using a comfortable hands-free headset. Not only do such phone calls provide a lifeline to the outside world and the people she misses, but they also serve as a distraction from the pain.

"The support of friends is crucial to enjoying life with chronic illness, so I go out of my way to make sure I can hang out with my friends as often as possible," Jenni says. This requires adopting several proactive approaches that better guarantee her plans will be successful in spite of her symptoms. If she knows an important gathering is coming up, she's extra diligent about resting the day before to conserve energy. She often eliminates strenuous physical activities before the event so "trouble spots" like her feet and hips don't flare up, especially since parties and dining events often entail long periods of time spent in uncomfortable chairs that strain joints anyway. Sometimes she'll bring another pair of shoes that are more comfortable, or use her back pillow to help alleviate the stress of hard chairs, and she doesn't demur when it comes to asking a friend for his or her seat if she's been standing for a long time and just needs to rest for a bit.

The steps Jenni implements are neither difficult to attain nor hugely inconvenient for her or anyone around her. However, they do indicate a level of forethought and awareness of her body's needs that doesn't happen overnight, and simple things like resting before an event or bringing more sensible shoes make a notable difference in terms of quality of life. In the end, individual preference and disease-specific needs dictate the types of things we do to make sure we're still social. We can't control every aspect of our conditions, but recognizing what we can do differently is crucial if we want to be fair, both to our bodies and the people we care about most.

32.

THE BIG "E"

Muster empathy, not exasperation

Our chronic illnesses may make us more empathetic toward others with illness, but that does not necessarily carry over to our responses to healthy people when they happen to be sick. From co-workers, everyday acquaintances, and classmates to good friends and loved ones, the people in our lives are bound to be felled by a cold, virus, or other temporarily incapacitating condition at some point. Since we've all been subject to the miseries of sinus congestion, the aches of fevers, and the general malaise of infection, we know how they're feeling. But does that mean it's always easy to listen—or that it's always easy for them to talk to us about it?

Personally, I think it's the people who are closest to us and know many of the details we may keep hidden from public view who have the biggest stake in the ongoing quest for mutual empathy. After all, it's only natural to turn to friends when something's wrong, and it's only natural that friends want to be able to do or say something helpful and supportive. But once the element of perspective is added to this seemingly obvious friendship equation, the situation isn't as uncomplicated as we'd like to believe.

One day I was on the phone with a good friend of mine who was recovering from a sinus infection. Though she was on the mend, her voice still sounded a bit nasal and I could tell her head was probably pounding from the congestion. She excused herself once to cough, and after a muffled few seconds, she returned to the phone.

She then made fun of her cough, saying it was nothing compared to mine. She'd been privy to some of my marathon twelve-hour coughing jags in the past, and I imagined she had one of those scenes in her head as she spoke. She sounded sheepish.

"Don't be silly. You still sound pretty miserable and have every right to say so," I told her, and I meant it. A cold is annoying and incapacitating no matter how healthy you are otherwise.

We moved on to other things—plans for the weekend, a mutual friend's engagement, my puppy's latest shoe massacre—but her comment lingered in my mind for several days. It wasn't the first time I'd had such a conversation, but this time I really noticed how chronic illness influenced even the most basic interactions with people. What troubled me the most was that I didn't ever want to become a martyr for my illnesses, nor did I want them to affect the balance of give and take that exists in any good relationship. I've come to re-alize that the source of our mutual discomfort that day on the phone is the fact that the healthy and the sick have competing rights to compassion and empathy.

Usually I know what to say and do when people I know don't feel well, have a complaint about a doctor or hospital, or are worried about an upcoming appointment. In these instances, it's actually a positive that I have spent my life in and out of doctors' offices and labs, because when I nod my head in commiseration and say things like "I totally hear you, that's so annoying," they sense true understanding of their particular grievances.

But there are times when I am worn out from my illnesses or overloaded trying to catch up on missed work and I just do not have the additional energy or inclination to be empathetic. I cannot deal with problems that, in the moment, seem so minor compared with mine. That commiseration, that understanding of similar situations and emotions, isn't there. I am stuck in one place—fear, frustration, disappointment—and I can't relate to other people. Or won't relate, to be more accurate.

After dealing with pain for more than ten years, Jenni also has days when the realities of her illness can bog her down a bit. "It's been one third of my life that I've dealt with this on a daily level. I've accepted it and know it will be always be there, but there are some days where I still say, 'Goddammit' and have a little pity party for myself," she says. Days like that are especially hard when she's confronted with friends with a cold or some other minor illness. The inclination to mourn particular losses and feel resentment in these types of situations is inevitable. "You can't live in that space, but everyone needs a moment," she says.

You know what it's like: As soon as you're well enough to leave your little cocoon, you bump into people at work near the copy machine, in hallways outside conference rooms or seminar halls, or at the bar waiting to order a drink, and suddenly you're confronted with their complaints. The banter is innocent and innocuous—it is meant to be innocent and innocuous—and yet inside you feel like exploding. This is the ugly side of chronic life. During those instances when I cannot be the type of friend I should be, I still smile and nod in the right places and murmur expressions of concern. I do what I need to do to keep the natural rhythm of conversation and the expected flow of information going—I ask how long they've been feeling sick or if they think they'll be able to take a break from work soon and recharge a bit—but even though I say the right things, it doesn't mean I always feel them.

When my turbulent health settles down and I regain my genuine empathy for the temporary suffering of my healthy family, friends, and co-workers, I always regret those instances of resentment. No one has a market on suffering. Though our perspectives are often quite different, the healthy and the sick are entitled to the same empathy and understanding from others when times are difficult. Of course what we each define as a "tough time" is always going to be relative, but that's exactly the point: suffering is determined by the sufferer, not by the observer. When people tell us they are having a tough time, we should try to be supportive friends or earnest listeners.

33.

GUILT: THE ULTIMATE DEAL-BREAKER?

*Being fair to friends is hard; figuring
out what fair means for significant
others is even harder*

I F THERE IS ANY EMOTION so replete in the experience
of living with chronic illness that it attaches itself to almost every kind of circumstance or relationship, it is guilt.
This is true in matters of the heart, especially as we get
older and our relationships become more serious. For some
people, illness is a deal-breaker. Despite the many examples
in this book where this is clearly not the case, there are certainly people who would consider chronic, serious, or terminal illness as a reason to back out of a relationship.

Brian turns this conventional notion on relationships on
its head, for the older he gets and the more he thinks about
his future, the more *he* considers his own CF a deal-breaker.
"It's partly because I am sicker now. But now that people are
getting older, in their midtwenties and thirties, you also sort

of can't help but think about [a long-term commitment]," he says. He's right—if you're his age and you're not interested in casual relationships, how can you *not* worry about how your condition would affect a long-term partner?

Usually when we talk about getting older in relation to dating, we're referring to women who want to get married and have children or have children without getting married, before it's too late. They reach a certain age and don't want to date casually anymore out of fear they are wasting time. Ours is a culture where the business of weddings spawns television series and mass hysteria, and in some circles, freezing eggs for use later in life is a commonplace conversational topic. Brian's point of view is different because he asks the very question that is so fundamental and so difficult to ask without flinching: If you really love someone that much, how could you ask that person to go through all of this?

For Brian, a seminal event in his perspective on relationships occurred when he was a teenager, in love with a wonderful girl who did not seem troubled by his having CF. In fact, things were going so well that he wanted to introduce his girlfriend to his lifelong CF doctor. During his trip to the hospital, he visited a good friend of his, someone he'd always looked up to as a mentor and a guide, someone who formed the backbone of the CF community Brian had grown up with in the hospital. His friend had recently gotten married, and Brian had high hopes for the couple's future—until he saw his friend, and realized he was dying.

"He'd just gotten married, yet he looked like he'd been beaten to death. He was so skinny he looked like a Latino Holocaust survivor. He could barely look at me," Brian says. Then he looked at his friend's wife, the stricken expression on her face as she tried to avoid meeting his eyes, and that moment was punctuated by two overwhelming feelings: survivor's guilt that he was doing so well and his friend was dying, and a growing understanding that someone might have that same stricken look of concern for him someday.

Brian was reminded of this moment and the look on that young wife's face a few years later when his girlfriend at the time, who had been accepting and open about his CF, watched him get an IV inserted in the hospital. "I saw it in her face, a mixture of fear and pity. She had these sad doe-eyes," he says.

He's always been someone who loved deeply and without reservation, someone who admits he "loves being in love," but his attitude about dating has changed as have his expectations and awareness of his CF. He admits that part of him is resigned to never having the family he's always wanted or being with someone long-term, because if he loved someone that much, he's not sure he could set her up to experience the inevitable pain of his disease progression. He hasn't found a solution; even now, he discusses a fledgling romance, and despite his happiness, he also alludes to difficult conversations in the near future.

Brian has dared to ask himself the question that many patients with serious illnesses tuck into the recesses of their minds, the question they know is there but is not easy to address. However, an equally pertinent corollary to the question consuming so much of Brian's thoughts about relationships is this: As patients, is it fair of us to make such decisions for other people? Aren't questions of risk and loss and unpredictability part and parcel of opening yourself up that deeply?

In Brian's case, every girl he has dated has known about his CF from the start and has been involved in had candid discussions about it. If a woman is well informed and realistic about his future and chooses to proceed, should her acceptance of these risks be enough to assuage his guilt? He's had girlfriends tell him to give them some credit, that it's their choice to be present in the relationship, but questions of choice and fairness are always colored in his mind by the fact that he has seen what this kind of loss looks like and they have not. Always his own devil's advocate, he still tempers these thoughts with the equally compelling point that anyone can die at any time—what if he didn't die of CF but instead got run over by a car? Would that loss be any less painful. Would the risk of loving have been less worth taking?

In the end, there is no one piece of sage advice Brian, I, or any other patient can offer that resolves this conflict between guilt and fairness. Patients deserve the same kinds of meaningful relationships healthy people strive for, and the people who love them deserve the choice to stay in a relationship with them or not. Of all the challenges and conflicting sentiments and questions of obligations and limitation implicit in living with chronic illness, this is one of the toughest ones to tackle. The only thing I can say is that guilt is a powerful, pervasive force whose influence in our relationships only grows larger when we refuse to acknowledge it.

34.

THE "OTHER" RELATIONSHIP-
DEFINING TALK

*Being candid about illness can only
expose the truth about your
relationship*

L IKE MOST TWENTYSOMETHINGS, I wanted to be exciting and energetic, not pale and run-down. Surrounded by the high heels and hardened nails of the young professionals who flocked to the Boston bars my friends and I went to on weekends, I suddenly felt very out of the loop and very tired. It was during this time that I was in and out of the hospital frequently and in the middle of all the tests and procedures that would eventually result in my diagnoses of PCD and bronchiectasis. I felt like I was living two lives: In one, I wore hospital gowns, produced sputum into a cup, and had discussions weighing issues of disease mortality versus disease morbidity. In the other, I wore jeans with heels, straightened my curly hair, and pretended I was just another recent grad surviving on laughably low wages and sour-apple martinis—as long as I kept the details of the "other" life to myself.

The façade was an exhausting ruse to maintain, and I can pinpoint the exact moment when I strayed off course. I met my now-husband, John, at the coat check of the downtown bar where my roommate and I hosted a New Year's Eve party. He was a foot taller than me, and his shockingly blue eyes somehow managed to look kind, even in the murky lighting of the subterranean bar. We chatted briefly, exchanging typical introductions and discussing the mutual friends. Hours later, we found each other again, just in time for the midnight kiss.

Earlier that day I doubted I would even be well enough to attend the party. I had been released from the hospital just two days earlier. I'd spent both Christmas and Thanksgiving in the hospital that year, and if there was ever a time when I was more interested in recovery than romance, it was then.

"What happened to your arms?" John asked as we moved from the edge of the crowded dance floor to talk. I pulled at my wrap, which had slipped down around my elbows. My arms were trailed with deep purple bruises, remnants of collapsed veins from IV insertions.

Bolstered by a glass of champagne on an empty, medicine-filled stomach and weary of the act I'd perpetuated all night, I did something that would normally horrify me: I told him upfront that I was sick.

"I was in the hospital recently because I have a lung disease and had an infection. They're just from the IVs," I said, pointing to the bruises.

I have to admit, part of my decision to be forthright also stemmed from the fact that I didn't want him to think they were track marks, a frequent joke among my friends. Sick was one thing; junkie was another beast altogether.

"Oh wow. Are you okay?"

"Well, yeah. Okay enough to be here, anyway. Especially after all the planning I did for it."

"Oh . . . But I mean are you *okay*? What's wrong?"

I almost laughed, because at the time, that was sort of the million-dollar question in my life. We were pretty sure it was PCD, but pending another lung biopsy, it wasn't conclusive yet, so for the time being, I was still the girl who coughed a lot and provided lots of questions for people but had few answers for them.

"It's kind of a long story. Basically, I have a chronic disease that's sort of similar to cystic fibrosis," I said.

He nodded in familiarity. "Is it serious?"

I was definitely letting this conversational train derail further by the second. The enormity of my disclosure cut through the champagne haze.

"Well, I don't know. I guess. But not too bad; I mean, I'm here, right?" I asked, and tried to steer the conversation to more normal topics. I think I even commented on the weather, which, given the predictable chill of New England winters, was a sign of my rising panic. What can you say about winter in Boston that is remotely interesting? That it's cold?

Burned in the back of my mind were the words a friend said to me when I was in high school: "Thinking of your life stresses me out. I can't do this." The comment was still damaging enough to haunt me years later, especially during major points of transition in my life. Why would someone new want to get involved with me when there were plenty of healthy people around? John asked for my number, but I didn't believe he'd actually call.

I've joked about the fact that John and I never had the "RDT"—relationship-defining talk—because we were so obviously exclusive from the start that it would have been redundant. But my joke isn't totally accurate—what was our very first conversation, if not in some way relationship-defining? From the beginning, John knew I was sick. He didn't know the intricacies of my conditions and he couldn't begin to know the many ways my illnesses would later impact his life, but he made the decision to ask for my number and then take me out on a date knowing I wasn't healthy. I'm not saying illness defined our relationship then or that it wholly defines it now, certainly. But because the truth was out there so early, a truth that would make some people hesitant, we didn't have to waste time keeping up pretenses or darting around important discussions.

While John and I had the initial uncomfortable illness discussion extremely early—to this day, I am grateful for the honesty that exhaustion and champagne conspired to give me—the "sick talk" is never easy, no matter when it happens. Jade finds that it is when boyfriends or potential romantic interests see her experience a severe pain flare for the first time that problems can arise. Until they witness the manifestation of her condition firsthand, they have no real basis for understanding chronic pancreatitis or what it means to live with it—it simply doesn't seem real, or like something that will in any way impact them. Yet she cannot hide these episodes, because they speak to a fundamental truth about her life that isn't going away. When confronted with it, the men she's dated oftentimes want to "fix it" or, realizing it is not something that is fixable, they get scared. Compounding this is the fact they sometimes take it to heart when she makes plans and then has to cancel them unexpectedly because she doesn't feel well, a phenomenon anyone with chronic conditions can attest has the potential to cause strife in relationships. Though she did date someone a few years ago who was wonderful during a bout of hospitalizations and flares—visiting her constantly and helping to care for her—in her experience, this type of situation is relatively uncommon.

In Vicki's case, she didn't have many obvious symptoms of her cystic fibrosis until her midtwenties, so she could cultivate her own sense of denial about being sick without her body giving her secrets away. As long as she looked young and fit and healthy to someone else, then perhaps she wasn't really as sick as her diagnosis suggested.

Reflecting on the men in the relationships where she didn't disclose her CF status, she says, "It wasn't them. It was that I wasn't comfortable enough with myself." Her words bring me back to my own fears, and she's right— until you are comfortable with your own identity and your own prognosis, there's no way you can be comfortable sharing that identity. Considering the fact that I went so long without even knowing the definitive cause of my illnesses, it makes sense to me that I was so diffident about owning them. At the same time, even though Vicki had always known exactly what was wrong with her, the marked changes in her condition when she reached her midtwenties made her CF status something much more uncomfortable and painful.

In the past, Vicki had always been able to pass off her frequent cough as bronchitis or something else benign, but after a few months of dating her now-husband, Dan, it became more and more conspicuous. Her moment of disclosure (her "RDT") came one night when they went to see *Mamma Mia!* Dan turned to her at one point and asked, "Are you always going to have that cough?"

Vicki knew it was time to be honest with him, and the vulnerability of that moment was excruciating.

"*Please* do not go home and look CF up on the Internet," she begged him, knowing that much of the material out there was negative and that it might be hard for him to realize that each case was different and one person's progression has little bearing on someone else's. Would he be able to look at her the same way once he knew the reality of her life?

Dan did go home and read everything he could find about cystic fibrosis right away—who wouldn't?—but afterward, he and Vicki were able to start a dialogue about illness, one that focused on integrating her illness into their relationship, and they became more serious. As it turns out, the truth doesn't cloud relationships; our own ability to process that truth enough to live with it does.

35.

THE SICKNESS STANDARD

*Like it or not, chronic illness takes
the ambiguity out of relationships*

NONE OF THIS IS EVER GOING AWAY, John. Sure you
don't want to be with someone healthy?" I asked
him, half teasing. It was the day after I'd undergone a lung
biopsy, about two months into our relationship. The sur-
geons had inserted a GI probe while I was under anesthesia,
so two wires from a monitor strapped around my waist
were taped to the side of my face and threaded down my
nasal passage, through my esophagus, and finally into my
stomach. I had to wear the probe for forty-eight hours to
see if irregularities in my GI tract were contributing to my
breathing problems. It was an awkward contraption, and
just as I finished speaking, I sneezed. Because of the tubes, I
couldn't control it well and a bloody mess spewed out of
my nose and onto my shirt. I looked down at the mess and
up at John.

"Sexy, huh?" I asked, completely mortified.

"Unbelievably," he said with a laugh, and set about cleaning me up, easing me out of the soiled shirt and gingerly pulling a clean one through the tubes and over my head.

This illustrates that illness can serve as a poignant litmus test, especially since people with chronic illness don't often have the luxury of carefree dating. Dating is simply more complicated—no less wonderful, thrilling, or incredible, of course—when chronic illness is present. Whether it's navigating embarrassing bodily fluids, looking at needles and injections, or massaging away frequent pain, chronic illness has an intrinsic ability to weed out the fainter of heart. In addition to the weightier issues of mortality and morbidity, illness can also be messy, dirty, phlegmy, smelly, sweaty, and anything but appealing, and the more corporeal aspects of it are equally telling. After all, if someone can find you attractive even when you've got a GI probe shoved down your nose and are covered in blood and snot, that someone is likely in it for the long haul.

Being sick can make you vulnerable enough, but with some diseases, the symptoms and side effects themselves can make romantic relationships that much more daunting. "CF isn't even an attractive disease. There's the gross cough, the foul-smelling stools—it's really just disgusting sometimes," Vicki says. Dan hardly seems to notice any of that. Obviously he hears her cough and he worries about her and is as vigilant about her health as she is, but the more unpleasant sounds and smells barely register with him. Now that she has a feeding tube coming out of her stomach, because CF can inhibit the body's ability to absorb nutrients, Vicki feels especially self-conscious. To her seeming amazement, her husband finds her as attractive as ever. "He'll look at me sometimes and say to our infant son, 'You have a sexy mama,' " she says. "I guess that's love, because I don't know how else he could still feel that."

John handled the sneeze fiasco and the lung biopsy itself with aplomb. He'd spent little time in hospitals, and there he was, spending the day in the waiting room with my parents, whom he'd only met once, and seeing me drugged and hooked up to oxygen. That's a lot to deal with when you've only known someone for a few months. He didn't blink at the assorted cups sitting around my apartment for me to spit in when I had a productive cough, and he didn't flinch at extended discussions of bowel obstructions and enemas, medications that smelled like rotten eggs, or the reactions to certain meds that caused me to vomit loudly and frequently in the next room.

Dating me sounds like it was an awesome time, huh? Yet he hung in there, he washed my face and inspected the color of my phlegm, he did my chest PT, and he listened to the "whales" in my chest with a stethoscope. I had no way of knowing that spring that we would get engaged only a few months later, but I did know that this was a guy who wasn't simply dating me to pass the time. He had invested his mind and his heart in me, despite some pretty unappealing circumstances.

Obviously no one illness has the market on visceral and visual indicators of illness. Kerri fielded questions about her insulin pump the very first night she met her now-fiancé, Chris, and whether it's when she's in a bathing suit or figuring out where it will go when she puts on her wedding dress, the pump is ever-present in their relationship, a three-dimensional representation of the role her diabetes plays in their lives. As they became closer, Chris witnessed things like the shaky, sweaty nighttime blood sugar lows, the kind that drenched their sheets and made her shiver. In Jenni's case, her fibromyalgia was diagnosed close to the time she met the man she would marry, so chronic pain, fatigue, and many lifestyle adjustments became an unavoidable part of his vocabulary as well.

Beyond the immediate physical litmus test, chronic illness clarifies motivations and potential in relationships like few other things can. For example, as Vicki and Dan's relationship continued to progress, there was no way CF could remain on the periphery. With any type of serious or life-threatening illness, you can't think of the long term without thinking about projected lifespan, you can't abstractly discuss marriage without thinking about how soon it should happen, you can't think about children in theory without discussing the practical associated risks and difficulties. I can't imagine that once you know you love someone and he or she loves you back, you would waste much time at all, especially if you are getting to the point in your life when you want marriage and children. Like Vicki's therapist told her when she was grieving the loss of her job and her professional identity, her life would inevitably become about her relationships. If Dan factored more and more in her life, then CF had to factor more and more into his as well.

Even a few years into their marriage, Vicki can't help but notice the difference in tenor between her and Dan's conversations and those of most couples she knows. Their friends might worry about the cost of living, paying the bills, or where they should go for dinner, but Vicki and Dan have always had to worry about, say, if they will be able to grow old together, or more recently, if they can join their friends on vacation, because she is on the lung transplant list and can't be far away from home in case she gets the call that her team has found lungs for her.

We put up with a lot on account of our illnesses—

embarrassing moments, scary moments, difficult moments. Anyone who is going to become part of our lives has to face the same moments with us. The constant presence of illness challenges relationships, but in the end, those challenges remove the ambiguity from our relationships and the challenge is well worth it.

36.

MELTDOWN MODE

*Sometimes the little nuisances of
illness can serve as the tipping point*

IT WAS A CONTAINER OF HONEY mustard salad dressing that turned out to be my Waterloo, the moment of
my crushing, flabbergasting defeat. I knew I would reach
my personal breaking point eventually, and I suspected that
it would likely concern something small and insignificant,
but even I was shocked at the turmoil of what will forever
be called the Honey Mustard Meltdown in our home. I
think John still quivers a bit inside whenever I order it.

It was a cold Friday night in November, the kind of
forlorn evening that begs for warm comfort food and thick
pajamas. John and I had been running errands for several
hours, and even before we left the house I'd been hungry and
tired. On Fridays I am usually exhausted from the usual
grind of work and fatigue anyway, but I'd been battling an
infection all that week and had yet to find the right combination of medicine to improve my peak flow readings and

cut down on my cough, so that day I was more worn out than normal. By the time we'd placed an order for take-out at nine P.M., I was way past the hunger stage and well into the ornery stage. Because of my celiac disease, the only option for me at the neighborhood pizza joint was salad, which, under normal circumstances, is perfectly fine with me. I ordered my usual—Greek salad with grilled chicken and honey mustard dressing on the side—but I had no desire to eat it. I was starving, freezing, and grumpy, and for once I wanted to have what I actually felt like eating, not what I *had* to eat. The smell of garlic and pizza crust was overwhelming, and only fueled my wallowing. The one beacon of light in my annoyed little world was the honey mustard dressing, which I've had an irrational obsession with for the past few years.

We circled around for a parking spot, lugged the shopping bags in, and settled down for dinner. I took the salad out of the bag, turned off by the limp greens and flaccid chicken. I was still somewhat hopeful as I reached in for my tangy, sweet salvation, but when I pulled the container out of the bag and pried off the lid, instead of the expected gooey goodness, I found watery, pungent Greek dressing.

I burst into tears. In a fit of rage, I flung the entire salad and the offending dressing into the trash.

"Are you serious with this? It's just dressing," said an understandably confused John. I know he thought I was being unbelievably immature.

"It's not about the dressing. It's everything. All I want is for something to be simple and uncomplicated for once. I didn't even want the stupid salad, I am so sick of salad, but if I have to have it, then is it too much to ask for the dressing to be what I wanted? I mean, is it really that hard to put the right container in the bag?" I screamed. Between my frustration and the fact that I hadn't eaten in over nine hours, I was now shaking.

"Laur, you gotta calm down. It's not worth this. Do you want me to order something else? Do you want me to cook something?"

By now, I was far too invested in my tantrum to consider being reasonable. I turned him down and stormed into the bedroom, where I proceeded to sob into the pillows. I was acting childish and I knew it, but I didn't care. It was easier to shut the door and cry than it was to try to explain how on this particular night, the crappy Greek dressing symbolized all the tiny little aggravations that had accumulated over the years.

John admires how cool and unflappable I can be in the serious, life-threatening moments, the way I handle bad news, painful procedures, or equally stressful medical events without getting emotional or losing control. But like many healthy people, he finds it hard to understand why it can be the little things, the trivial setbacks and inconveniences, that momentarily blindside me. I've read that people with serious illness "don't sweat the small stuff" and other trite platitudes in all sorts of essays and confessionals, and I have to say, I don't buy it. Not all the time, anyway. Maybe there are patients out there who can be so serene, so sensible and enlightened at every moment, but I'm not one of them. I'm tough, but meltdown mode is just as real as maintenance mode in my life.

Despite our best efforts and diligence in taking care of the daily demands of illness, many of the larger issues are sometimes out of our grasp. I can take all my medications, comply with my physical therapy, get regular exercise and enough sleep—all the machinations of rudimentary control—but in the end, when an infection is bad enough or an exacerbation serious enough, I have no control over what happens. As a result, it becomes even more important to me to control the small things, the details I can predict. When even those seemingly innocuous details don't go right, I feel completely helpless. In the moment, I cannot be articulate or philosophical about it, and so my anger and my frustration speak for me: *Why can't anything be simple?*

I doubted the healthy people in my life realized just how much thought and planning went into so many routine activities, and was frustrated with myself for even caring about that. I viewed all this medical minutiae, this endless weighing of options and benefits, as one more thing other people couldn't understand. The more niggling details I had to consider, the more grimly determined I was to make sure nothing escaped my control.

Like all lifelong patients, I'd always had to worry about the details—packing my medications when I went to sleep over a friend's house, bringing my inhalers to gym class, using my nebulizer before school in the morning—from a very young age. So why did it suddenly seem so much more consuming, and why was the threat of something going awry so much more palpable? There are logical, intellectual explanations. First, my health status had deteriorated over the years—certainly the increase in hospitalizations that marked each year since high school were evidence of that. With additional problems and treatment plans came additional considerations. Second, by the time we're in our twenties, we've naturally accumulated more of the usual age-appropriate responsibilities and more-significant relationships; as our lives become more complicated, so do our chronic concerns.

Of course, my family had already prepared me for the rigors of negotiations, compromises, and above all else, complications: My father juggles chemo infusions around his busy work schedule, carries his insulin needles in the breast pocket of his suit coat, and never goes anywhere without a little insulated lunch bag stocked with apples, juice, and a turkey sandwich in case his blood sugar gets low. My mother needs pillows to sit in most chairs, and whenever she leaves the house for more than a couple of hours, she makes sure she has her heating pad, her TENS unit (a device that pulsates her shoulders and calms down nerve pain), and ready access to ice. They'd been living like this for so long they no longer have to think about it, and at times I felt guilty that I can't say the same thing of myself.

And yet I know they each have their own breaking points too. For my mother, it usually involves cleaning or cooking: the kitchen isn't clean enough, the rearrangement of her closet doesn't work out the way she'd planned, the home-delivery grocery service hasn't gotten the order right. Depending on the day, the woman who can withstand searing electrical pain and endure bone spurs the size of small oranges attacking her joints can be brought down by things of much less significance. As for my father, he doesn't complain about the nausea from chemo, the shaky lows and fuzzy highs of diabetic blood sugar swings, or the pain in his muscles when his connective tissue disease flares. But the older he gets, the less tolerance he has for things that require patience: routine traffic sends him cursing, lines at stores can be so frustrating that he'd just as soon leave than purchase his desired item, and if instructions for electronic gadgets are more than one page long, he's been known to toss both gadget and instructions into a drawer or a closet, never to be seen with again. It's just another frustration.

Does that mean both of them aren't strong? Certainly not. Does that mean they don't belong to the tribe of people who "don't sweat the small stuff," or some equally pedestrian saying? Not at all. But it does mean that, like me, they reach a point where they're too fed up with the daily skirmishes with illness to have tolerance for much else. Healthy people may not get this, but speaking from the perspective of a girl who withstood twenty-five surgeries by age fourteen but was felled by the wrong salad dressing, it makes a lot of sense to me. I am as sheepish about meltdown mode as I am annoyed by it, but once the tears have stopped and sanity has again returned, I recognize its place in the complicated system of checks and balances that is living with chronic illness—and I think John does too.

37.

WALKING THE LINE

*You may be an illness expert, but
don't forget your significant other
is still learning*

O NE OF THE HARDEST THINGS for our loved ones
and friends to get used to is trusting us enough to let
us follow our instincts and knowledge. In the healthy world,
when there is a problem, the doctor has the final say. If I lived
like that, I would spend nearly every day calling the doctor or
going to the hospital. Intuition has a much larger role in my
life and my health. My body is a sneaky and demanding
teacher, but after so many years, I have learned from it. I've
yielded to it when necessary, and dismissed it when possible.

I know the second I wake up whether the tightness in my
chest is simply because I need to loosen up anything that
may have settled in my lungs overnight or whether it's the
tightness that accompanies the beginning of an infection.
The latter feels just the tiniest bit *colder*. I can tell by how
hard I can press on my quad muscle before I flinch from

pain if my legs are just sore from exercise or if it will be a "bad" day for my adrenalitis and fatigue and I won't be able to move my legs by lunchtime. If it's the latter, I must plan ahead so as not to get trapped wherever I am when the total shutdown occurs. Perhaps most important, when I fill up with phlegm and begin coughing and wheezing spasmodically, I can tell within two to three minutes if it is an episode I will be able to contain with my meds and equipment at home or if I need to go to the hospital. Making the decision to self-medicate or head for the hospital before my oxygen saturation is too low and my airways are too constricted can literally mean the difference between life and death, or moderately aggressive treatment versus intubation, so those minutes are essential, and I know my limits.

Was it reasonable to expect John would draw the same boundaries?

I think this was the most difficult part for him, being torn between his knee-jerk reaction to seek help when he saw me gasping for air and his desire to trust my judgment. I imagine it's the same mix of fear and understanding most people experience when learning to trust other people's judgments, the same flux Chris must have felt when he first watched Kerri treat a blood sugar low with juice and wondered if it would be enough, the same desire Dan must have had to do something to stop Vicki's especially severe coughing jag, even though intellectually he knew coughing helped clear her lungs. At its core, this experience has less to do with sick people's expertise versus healthy people's expectations and more to do with the basic human instinct to want to do something to alleviate the suffering in others. Chronic patients simply have different thresholds and tolerances for symptoms that would typically invoke worry or distress in otherwise healthy people.

In the beginning of our relationship, every time my breathing deteriorated to a critical point, John would want to rush to the hospital. If I had to watch him struggle to breathe and I wasn't used to that, I know I'd react in much the same way. I now wince at my harshness, but I finally jolted him into seeing my perspective: "Listen," I told him, "I don't have a death wish, you know. When I need to go, no matter how much I hate it, I will always go. Trust me when I say I will let you know when I need to, okay?" It was late spring, a few months into our relationship, and I knew things with John were serious. I needed to know he could trust me to be the best judge of my health.

And he listened. Or, I should say, listens. I know it isn't easy for him, but he lets me make the call and does not question me nearly as much. One night shortly before we got engaged we drove the hour's trip from the Providence, Rhode Island, airport to Boston. I felt things were off in my chest. I had been coughing more than normal all day, and things got too tight in my chest too quickly.

"There is an elephant sitting on my chest right now, John. It's squashing the air right out of me," I said when it first started. "It doesn't feel right. Something's going to happen."

With twenty minutes left in the ride, my chest almost completely closed up, to the point where I was too tight to even cough up any phlegm or even wheeze; all I could do was gasp for air. It was dark and rainy that night, and I gripped the door handle as I tried to slow down my breathing, unsuccessfully attempting to match my inhalations with the steady, rhythmic pace of the windshield wipers.

"What do you want to do? I can bring you right to the hospital, or we can get home and try your neb and try to get some of this stuff up, Laur. Your call," he said calmly, eyes focused on the slick pavement ahead of him.

"Just . . . *gasp* get me . . . *gasp* home. We'll give it . . . *gasp, gasp*,"—I paused to steady myself—"two nebs and see . . . *gasp, gasp* . . . if that cuts it . . . go from there . . ." I trailed off, exhausted from using that much air to speak.

He was perfect. He did not get flustered, did not panic, just got me home as quickly as possible, unlocked my door, and ran to set up the nebulizer. He clapped me while I positioned myself with the nebulizer mask and tubing, trying to manually break up the thick mucus that cut off my air supply. After a third nebulizer treatment for good measure, my lungs had opened up enough for me to cough up a lot of phlegm and the excruciating pain of the tightness had left.

"You did great, J. Thank you for trusting me and not rushing me to the ER automatically."

"Hey, I'm learning, you know? It's still as scary to me, but not as new, so I expect that you know what to expect."

I hugged him, thinking to myself, "Now this is a partner. Not just a life partner, but a health partner. He listens to my body as I listen to my body."

It's a learning curve that continues to evolve. I find that the more he trusts my assessment of my body's needs, the more comfortable I am in seeking out his opinion and trusting his assessment as well.

38.

PARTNERS IN HEALTH

*Don't be afraid to be vulnerable—it's
the best way to show strength*

W HEN JOHN FIRST ASKED TO LEARN how to do my
chest physical therapy, I was pleasantly surprised
and a little hesitant. I wondered if being this close to the
daily reality of illness would overwhelm him, and for me,
chest PT was the most telling constant reminder that I was
sick. Anytime we're involved in a romantic relationship,
there is often a specific action or process that is imperative
for our disease management and equally significant in terms
of our relationship's development. A partner's involvement
in treating conditions has been popularized in media and
culture more than ever before; even *Sex and the City* dab-
bled in the business of spousal intervention. Of course, the
scene where Trey injects Charlotte with fertility hormones
only touches the surface of the types of things people need
to be willing to do for chronic patients. However, this
glossy Hollywood depiction of the physical intrusions of

treatment or therapy still resonates: people we love often find themselves in the position of doing things that are at best uncomfortable and at worst extremely painful to us and for us.

"Am I doing this position right? I need to make sure I'm not smacking your kidneys when I'm doing the lower ones, right?" John asked on our fateful first chest PT session. It was a cold February day, almost two years since I'd graduated from college and eight months after I'd first started undergoing daily chest PT.

I strained to meet John's gaze as he struggled through the different positions. He was kneeling in front of the couch in my tiny living room in Beacon Hill. In addition to its ivy-covered brownstones, authentic gaslit streetlamps, ancient Brahmin wealth, and proximity to my graduate writing program at Emerson College, Beacon Hill had something else important to me: my new hospital, which was a mere thirty seconds from my apartment. In my postcollege quest for an accurate diagnosis, the number of appointments, tests, and hospitalizations made this closeness invaluable. I was lying on the couch on my right side, my stomach facing him. I had three pillows stacked under me at my waist so that my body formed an arc—head and legs curved down at each side, torso in the middle.

Clap! clap!

"You've got the right technique. Hear that sort of 'pop' when you hit? It means you're cupping your hands. But don't be afraid to hit harder—really whack me," I said.

John increased the pressure as he clapped the spot just beneath my armpit, one of eleven positions that target each lung lobe.

"Much better. You're a natural, you know. Most newbies just slap at me. Cupping is much harder," I continued.

I hoped the conversation would detract from the obvious bouncing of my breasts each time he made contact, despite the sturdiest of sports bras.

CLAP! *clap,* CLAP! *clap!*

John's rhythm was now a near perfect match to that of my regular therapist, Steve. Despite the cold draft, he'd already stripped down to his T-shirt, and now stopped to wipe a trickle of sweat off his brow. If you're not used to it, this pounding is hard work.

When John first surprised me by asking if he could learn how to do chest PT, we'd been dating a mere three weeks. It was long enough to know we were serious about each other, but not long enough for me to trust that meant illness and all. Sure, I'd uncharacteristically blurted out that I was sick when we first met, but telling him was one thing; I was still the gatekeeper and there were still all kinds of ways I could keep him separated from my illnesses. My "sick life," the daily chest PT appointments and medications, the almost weekly doctor's appointments—such trappings of illness were all things he wouldn't see or understand unless I chose to let him. Chest PT was what I guarded most, both because it was such a flagrant example of the medical institution's inextricable place in my life and because it was such a deeply personal and vulnerable process in a physical sense. Once John learned how to do chest PT, he wouldn't just be my boyfriend anymore, he would be a caregiver on an as-needed basis, and I wasn't sure I wanted that shift in our relationship to happen so soon.

At this point in our relationship, we'd survived both our first family function and our first real fight, and we had seamlessly evolved to the stage where we talked on the phone every single night, regardless of whether we'd just seen each other, without even realizing the pattern we'd established.

But all the while, I waited for the inevitable first medical crisis. Meeting my older brothers and a fight ostensibly spurred on by bad Thai take-out and two overtired, overworked people were natural milestones of a romantic relationship; emergency room visits and respiratory failure were certainly not. *What if the reality of all this is too much, too soon? Is this a mistake?* It didn't occur to me that in asking to learn how to care for me by doing chest PT, John had already accepted my reality. I can see now that allowing John to be part of something so intimate was much less about him seeing me as "weak" or "sick." I needed to see that it wasn't just about my feelings and emotions—only then could I appreciate the true issue at hand; the fact that he loved me enough to do something he knew was painful for me both physically and emotionally.

There are as many individual litmus tests and intimate processes as there are illnesses, and chest PT is only one example of this type of boundary crossing. For Kerri, who had lived with a definitive diagnosis for twenty years by the time she met her now-fiancé, Chris, diabetes was a part of the relationship from the beginning. Since Chris had limited experience with the disease, Kerri introduced the nuances of her condition step by step. Just as John became fluent in the names of medications and their particular side effects, Chris slowly became oriented to the particular language of diabetes. For example, he soon recognized what a blood sugar reading of 40 meant and automatically knew he should get Kerri some juice to help combat her "low."

But Kerri needed to know Chris could do something much more delicate than simply conversing in the jargon of diabetes or fetching her juice: he needed to be able to stick a needle into her should an emergency situation emerge where she needed a sugar shot and she was unable to do it herself.

The more comfortable and serious you get with someone, the more time you spend with that person. The more time you spend, the greater the likelihood that a chronic condition like diabetes and countless others will unexpectedly worsen when you're with that person. If he or she is going to be a significant part of your life, then it's crucial to know you can handle those types of situations together.

So Chris weighed the conflicting notion that what he did might hurt her with the fact that if he ever had to do it, it would really help her, and he practiced gingerly with an insulin syringe. "It was strange to watch someone stumble through what was so automatic for me after all these years," she says, a particularly valuable insight given the steep learning curve our significant others are often forced to adopt. Kerri may have been used to injecting herself without a second thought, but that didn't mean sticking a needle into his girlfriend was in any way easy or automatic for Chris.

This step in their relationship also yielded an even larger insight for Kerri—the fact that someone loved her enough to hurt her and loved her enough to get that scared created an usually close bond between them. She had someone who was willing to face her mortality with her and not look away. Though I didn't see it that day when I was instructing John on his rhythm and worrying about my sports bra, I'd found the same thing in him. Instead of feeling vulnerable and exposed, I ended up feeling incredibly secure and grateful I had a partner in my health.

39.

IN SICKNESS AND HEALTH

*Marriage prep courses don't tell you
how to be a chronic spouse—
experience does*

FROM WEB SITES LIKE theknot.com to bridal boot camp classes offered at my gym to pre-Cana classes for engaged couples in my parish, once John and I got engaged there were endless resources offering us some sort of preparation or education for planning a wedding, and more important, planning a marriage. My mother even gave me her yellowed copy of the *Better Homes and Gardens'* bride-to-be handbook she'd gotten from her own mother, a snapshot from a different era where meal plans involved ambrosia and dinnertime was synonymous with a skirt, heels, and a frilly apron.

John and I sorted through hotel packages and menus, we updated registries and made flight plans. We plowed through decisions like linen versus tulle, chocolate versus vanilla, and an evening ceremony versus an afternoon one. We also sorted through the heavy stuff in our marriage classes at church, discussing our feelings on faith, children, education, and spirituality. We made sure we were of like minds in terms of financial planning, lifestyle, and career trajectories. We even sat down and made an exhaustive spreadsheet of things to do for the wedding, complete with estimated dates of completion and relevant parties' contact information.

But what about the conversations on what it would be like being young and married with chronic illness? We didn't encounter those types of discussions on wedding sites, in church classes, or when we spoke with other engaged or married friends. Of all the relationship challenges and potential pitfalls the wedding sites and classes and bridal magazines warned about, this issue was perhaps the most defining and significant one to us.

So what would it take to make the shift from girlfriend to fiancée to wife in relation to illness? I'd gotten the role of "sick girlfriend" down well. There had been the initial hesitations when I wondered if my health would scare him away. There were also the revelatory moments when I realized I didn't mind being vulnerable with him. But I was used to being the one in charge of my health, whether that meant deciding to call the doctor or go to the hospital, deciding how many work-related projects to take on, or dealing with a new diagnosis. Suddenly, I needed to work John into this scenario, and I needed to break away from my habit of dealing with issues and making decisions on my own or with my parents, my longtime compatriots in all things illness. As my husband, he needed to be the one I turned to for this, just as I turned to him with everything else. I had to trust him with that last vestige of single-girl sickness protocol.

Illness is intensely personal and idiosyncratic, and each of us has developed our own ways of dealing with its many intrusions. If I were to run my own workshop to instill the basics of chronic marriage, my lesson plans would begin and end right here: Once you enter into a marriage or any type of long-term commitment, you have to be willing to let go of some of the very attitudes that have enabled you to survive and adapt to illness. It's never just about you anymore, or how you feel, how far you push yourself, or what decisions you make that may or may not be in your best interest. The same can be said about relationships in general, but chronic illness adds a whole other dimension to this notion since our physical health is so closely linked to the physical and emotional health of our loved ones.

No matter what precautions I take, I can't always control my conditions, but John understands my need to try. What I can do for both of us is remain diligent in following my treatment plan and taking my medications. I can be more realistic about the number of courses I teach a semester and how many freelance projects I accept. When I was single, the consequences of taking on too much were easier to contain, and also easier to dismiss or deny. It wouldn't be fair to wrap John up in the same maladaptive pattern now that we're married. I'd be lying if I said I didn't still briefly consider "jumping" at every opportunity that crosses my desk. Of course I do. I just don't blindly accept them anymore. I'm no longer on some sort of autopilot where I am incapable of seeing the ramifications of overextending myself on my health and my marriage.

40.

MARRIAGE BY NUMBERS

*Sick spouses can still maintain
healthy marriages*

THE U.S. DIVORCE RATE IN MARRIAGES where chronic illness is present is over 75 percent.[1] It's a number I've heard often in reference to illness and marriage. Seeing it once again made me stop and think about the demands chronic illness places on marriages, especially since I am only two years into a marriage that will forever be punctuated with sickness. What does it take to be in that elusive 25 percent of marriages that survive chronic illness, especially for younger couples?

Obviously, people divorce for all sorts of reasons, and there's not necessarily a causal relationship between chronic illness and divorce. But certainly between lost income due to sickness, high medical bills, loss of identity, pain, frustration, and so on, there are a lot of ways chronic illness could be implicated in these findings. "If there are problems in the marriage to begin with, the arrival of illness or disability can certainly help tip it over the edge," says Richard Anderson, president of the Well Spouse Association, an organization that supports spousal caregivers, and a veteran of what I've dubbed "chronic marriage."

"You just don't see a lot of literature that addresses chronic illness in younger marriages. It's so hard," says Jenni. She and her husband, Steve, have been married for five years, and the daily challenges of chronic illness, when considered in the long term, can sometimes seem overwhelming. "It's never going to go away; ten years later, are you still going to want to deal with all of it?" she asks, confronting the sometimes harsh reality of any chronic condition directly. And she is right—for however much research there is on the dynamics of marriage and long-term relationships and on illness and disability, very little research focuses on how illness affects younger couples and spouses.

The information that does exist confirms what all of us who live with these issues every day already know: illness often forces the healthy spouse to take on multiple roles—spouse, caregiver, breadwinner—and with more roles comes more stress and frustration and diminished marital quality. The following excerpt from the *Journal of Rehabilitation* does a good job of summing up the complexities of chronic marriages:

"Schumacher (1995) noted that, when a spouse assumes a caregiving role, there are many changes in the patterns of relating, and often each spouse must acquire new skills and insights. The impact of the illness or disability on the relationship between spouses and marital quality may be significant. Illness demands may expend family resources and affect the well spouse's perception of the marriage (Lewis, Woods, Hough, & Bensley, 1989). Both the well and the ill spouse may feel isolated while facing immense concerns.

Consequently, these tensions may exacerbate the stress of the illness. As Speziale (1997) described, even minor adjustments to chronic illness, in areas such as sexual intimacy or cognitive and emotional responses, may diminish closeness and cause strain in the relationship."[2]

Research about marriage also suggests that major contributors to marital quality for all couples include love, romance, physical intimacy, and communication.[3] All these factors are difficult to sustain on their own (you need only to consider the dismal divorce rate in our country as evidence of that fact), so imagine how much more difficult they are to nourish and develop when you add in the many pressures of illness, from the daily strain of not feeling well or feeling isolated to the fiscal repercussions of missing work and medical bills to the emotionally draining worries over mortality.

It's not something we linger over or obsess about, but John and I both know that we can never make any plans without thinking of the illness logistics, that whether it's planning Christmas dinner or a long-awaited weekend away, there is never an escape from illness. Even our wedding and honeymoon—easily the most fun, carefree, and joyous time in my life—were shaped somewhat by illness: the day of the ceremony was hot and humid, the air so sticky to breathe that we couldn't take any of the outdoor pictures we'd planned and the gluten-free top layer of the cake began to melt, despite the full-blast of the air conditioner. We spent many of our last hours in Napa Valley huddled on the couch in our suite while I used my nebulizer; by the time we got in the rental car and drove to San Francisco that afternoon, I had a full-blown fever and respiratory infection. John spent our first night in the city tracking down a Walgreens to refill an antibiotic prescription for me and we ate soup in our hotel room, marveling at the view of the city we wanted desperately to experience firsthand.

Don't get me wrong; our wedding day went smoothly and we had an absolutely amazing time. Our honeymoon was filled with good wine, good food, and beautiful sights. All of those things are true and illness did not eclipse them in any way. Considering there were moments in my life when I didn't think I'd live to get married, I viewed these minor inconveniences as merely white noise, static I could hear but nothing that came close to drowning out what was really important. My point is that there is no escape from illness. Most of the time, we don't mind this or don't even think about it. But there are days when it weighs us down, when it makes the normal toil and teamwork necessary for a marriage to survive even more pressing.

"It's all the things we have to deal with that other couples don't that is hard sometimes," Vicki says. In her case, the progression of her illness is reflected in the tenor of her conversations with her husband. Of course they have to think about all the little things like scheduling in chest physical therapy and getting jobs done around the house, but they also have so many larger issues to think about: her decision to put her name on the lung transplant list, what her timeline is and if they will have the chance to grow old together. These are not easy subjects to confront and acknowledge, but they are discussions Vicki and Dan cannot ignore, and they touch on realities that are deeply ingrained in their daily lives.

Sometimes I wish that all John and I had to worry about were the typical age-minded concerns of our peers: making mortgage payments, making appropriate career decisions, balancing work with social lives. I get sick of medications and infections and compromises, of even the simplest things being complicated. I worry because I know my "big" diseases—however stable and well controlled they are right now—are progressive, and I ask myself, "Is this as good as we're ever going to get?" Some days, I feel so positive and content with our lives that I don't mind answering that question; other days, it scares me to think about it.

With that niggling little 75 percent statistic in the back of our minds, where does all this information leave young couples dealing with chronic illness? Are we doomed to failure, our shot at success and happiness (or marital quality, to use the parlance of research) overshadowed by the significant stressors of illness?

Not a chance.

The longer I am married, the more I realize how fortunate I was to have grown up with sick parents. Obviously I'm not glad my parents aren't healthy, but as I stumble through the process of integrating my illnesses into our marriage, I recognize that the success of their thirty-five-year union is an invaluable resource for John and me. I always knew my parents' relationship was especially strong, but until recently I didn't realize how exceptionally rare it is—at least, according to the numbers. Maybe we can look at this from the complete opposite direction, and couples like John and me, and Vicki and Dan, and Jenni and Steve can comfort ourselves with the knowledge that for all its grief and complications, chronic illness can sharpen the very skills we need to survive as spouses, not as patients and caregivers. Because of illness, we don't have the luxury of avoiding difficult conversations, we're forced to be both completely trusting and completely vulnerable, and we know how to handle serious crises as a team. That's a fairly impressive skill set for a couple.

My parents married in their early twenties. At twenty-six, my father was first misdiagnosed as having muscular dystrophy, and their lifelong journey into the word of serious chronic illness began. For her part, my mother has also been sick for over two decades with severe arthritis and degenerative joint disease. So their relationship has been hit with illness on both sides. Yet with all the stress, the fear of death, the decades marked by setbacks and flares that few couples they knew had to contend with, they have a wonderful marriage. They have never had the luxury of simply worrying about "normal" things, and while they have stumbled under that burden from time to time, they have also used this knowledge to inspire each other.

My parents' marriage is an interesting example of caregiving: because both of them are sick, they take turns being the "healthy" one and doing things for the other. When my father is bedridden with an especially bad flare of his muscle disease or is worn out from his chemotherapy, my mother snaps to attention, taking care of plans and making sure he gets plenty of rest. When my mother is unable to do things around the house or loses several days in a row to the pain of her joint diseases, my father assumes control: the meals are cooked or bought, the refrigerator stocked, and endless cups of tea and ice packs are supplied for her. When someone you love is sick, you do what you need to do—it really does boil down to a statement as simple as that. John cancels his plans in order to sit with me on the couch. Dan takes care of their baby on weekends when Vicki isn't up to it. Steve understands when Jenni's chronic pain worsens and she isn't able to do the things they've planned.

"You do what you have to do, but you take on a lot," says Richard Anderson of the Well Spouse Association. After acting as a caregiver for more than thirty years, he feels that communication is the most important component of a lasting relationship. Clearly this is true for any relationship, whether illness is present or not, but when you consider the myriad challenges to marital equality and satisfaction chronic illness entails, its relevance is even more pronounced. In Richard's case, his wife was open and communicative about her epilepsy from the time they first started dating. When she was diagnosed with scleroderma after twelve years of marriage, she had been ill for some time and he already had a sense of what living with illness would be like. He knew a lot would be asked of him, but he was willing to do it for the woman he loved. Her diagnosis resulted in endless conversations: Was she up to the plans they'd made? Did she need him to take her to the hospital? Did he understand her decreasing interest in physical intimacy? Could he help her with her freelance writing and still take care of his own job? Without a mutual willingness to broach these often sensitive and painful areas—what is more private and irreplaceable than one's sense of independence or intimacy within a couple?—the stress and frustration illness caused could have driven them apart.

Turns out, the scant research available also supports what we chronic couples already know: many couples find their relationship is strengthened through their experiences with illness.[4] I can't find numbers for this, and I don't know how many marriages are quantifiably better or stronger for having no choice but to deal with illness. What I do have is empirical evidence, the shared experiences of the couples I have seen and talked to whose success is evident. Maybe the sicker you are, the more equipped you are to adapt when things don't go as planned. If you've faced nearly impossible odds and painful truths over and over and always manage to beat them, perhaps you begin to live with the knowledge that, together, you can handle just about anything. Perhaps, like my parents, you also learn that there is always room for hope and for growth, because in the darkest moments, that's all you have to cling to aside from each other.

41.

CARING FOR THE CAREGIVER

In chronic relationships, the
caregiver's needs are just as
important as the patient's

MY HUSBAND IS A SAINT," Vicki says. "I've never seen a man so selfless. He's top-notch, he literally waits on me hand and foot . . . but sometimes, I want to say, 'Stop being my nurse and just be my husband!' It drives me crazy because it's not something you can switch on and off."

Sound familiar? The tension between your spouse as life partner and your spouse as caregiver is emblematic of the many complexities of chronic marriages, and for as difficult as it can be to ask for help and be that vulnerable, it can be just as challenging to be the person always responsible for providing that help.

In Vicki's case, her husband is endlessly patient and supportive, and a few years into their marriage, the role of caregiver isn't one that overwhelms him. "My mother tells me that while God may have given me this illness, he also gave me this amazing husband," she says. But while Vicki is as grateful for her husband's constant support as he is willing to give it, this tenuous balance of multiple roles still has implications for their relationship. She bears a fair amount of guilt from what she perceives as her husband doing so much more for her than she does for him, a sentiment that resonates strongly with my own experiences and many of the patients I've encountered. It's a phenomenon that can cause significant strain in a relationship, and certainly something that should be part of any dialogue about what it's like to have your spouse also serve as your caregiver.

In our case, it's not uncommon for John to work full time, go to class or study groups after work, and then on the weekends do all the grocery shopping and cleaning because I am not up to helping him. We enjoy doing errands together, but by now we're both used to me fading in the middle of the store, completely drained of energy, and he knows he'll have to bring me home and finish the rest on his own. It doesn't always happen, and there are definitely times when I pick up the slack in terms of errands and household duties when he is especially busy with work, but I feel guilty when he's vacuuming and mopping and I'm on the couch. I feel frustrated when I've planned to make a nice dinner for him or promised to pick him up somewhere or meet him and I can't. I question the fairness of the situation for John, and wonder what I can do for him that would in any way compensate for all he does for me. As Vicki says of her own husband, "There's so much on his shoulders, he never gets a break."

Research suggests that spouses who take on the caregiver role—a role that ebbs and flows with the cyclic nature of chronic illness but never truly ends—are more likely to experience anxiety or depression than spouses who do not have the same responsibilities.[1] The same research also shows that people who are the long-term recipients of care from others also suffer from depression and low-self esteem as a result of the shift in marital equality and needing to rely on such help.[2] So the caregiver resents the extra burdens and the care recipient resents the fact that such help is necessary. It's important to distinguish that it isn't the person but the situation that causes resentment: when John gets frustrated or angry, he isn't angry with me; he's angry with the illnesses that get in our way. Similarly, when I get frustrated or overcome with a feeling of helplessness, I don't resent John's help or the fact that he is healthy and I am not; I resent illness for the things it takes away from me and from our relationship, that it puts me in the position of frequently needing help and John in the position of needing to give it to me.

Richard Anderson knows all too well the danger of burnout spousal caregivers face—his own experience with caregiver burnout is what initially led him to join the Well Spouse Association. For younger couples, the isolation and frustration often felt by spousal caregivers is further compounded by the fact that illness in younger couples is largely undervalued. "There's a stereotype out there that illness in couples is a senior citizens' thing. That's just not true! Twenty-three percent of family caregivers are spousal caregivers; nobody has even quantified how many spousal caregivers are under fifty-five," he says. As a result, people expect discussions about illness and coping when couples are elderly, but no one expects younger couples to have anything to say about it, so they remain shut off from the dialogue.

Richard cared for his first wife from the time they were newlyweds until she passed away over thirty years later. Early in the marriage, it was the social isolation that was especially difficult. "When you're young, you really notice that you lose friends. Chronic illness progresses and more complications set in, and people start to drift away. It's not deliberate, but it happens," he says. He emphasizes the unpredictable nature of chronic illness in this situation: most healthy young people are not familiar with these types of illnesses, and if people don't understand how sudden and drastically chronic conditions can change, it's extremely difficult to maintain friendships.

Throughout their marriage, as his wife's conditions worsened, more responsibilities fell on him. He describes a "rolling grief" that living with a chronically ill spouse incurs. He didn't notice changes on a day-to-day basis, but when he stepped back and looked at how much had changed gradually—the jobs and tasks his wife used to do but couldn't, the number of plans or trips they'd cancelled, the decrease in their physical intimacy, the increased time he spent doing things for her—he was stricken by the magnitude of the losses for each of them. "Fairly early on I learned to set really low expectations for what we could and would do so I wouldn't get upset if plans fell through," Richard says, remembering one time in their marriage when they'd invited friends over for drinks and he'd had to cancel the get-together at the last minute because his wife's symptoms flared. "I was so angry that illness was interfering with our lives," he says.

Over the years, the accumulated frustration and fatigue from juggling so many roles took its toll. Not only was he emotionally depleted and isolated, but he also developed type 2 diabetes after she died; he says instances where the "healthy" spouse begins to get sick from pushing too hard and doing too much for too long are not uncommon. "There needs to be a balance between looking after the sick spouse and looking after yourself. It's easy to go overboard and care for the other person and forget about your own needs," he says.

Richard brings up an especially poignant point: when you're the spouse of a sick person, when people call or visit, they always inquire about the patient. Rarely do people think to ask how the caregiver is, and that contributes to the isolation of healthy spouses. When I thought about this point, I realized how true it is. People call and ask how I am feeling all the time, but rarely does anyone think to ask John how he is doing with all of it—and I realized I needed to make a more conscious effort to do that too.

When Richard finally reached his personal breaking point, finding a support system like the Well Spouse Association was critical—not only did he find people he could talk to openly and honestly; he discovered there were people who felt just as isolated and frustrated by illness as he did. For obvious reasons, the sick spouse is the one who requires more attention and concern, but ignoring the physical and emotional needs of the caregiver is doubly dangerous—the caregiver runs the risk of becoming burnt out, and if that happens, the sick spouse suffers as well.

The most important thing in terms of navigating this caregiver–care recipient minefield is, unfortunately, often the hardest: communicating about it, honestly and openly. It was a year and half into our marriage before John admitted to me that sometimes he does get angry at the situation, namely his inability to make me well and his fears he is not doing enough for me. He didn't want to tell me because he thought it would hurt me.

"Of course it all gets to you at times," I told him. "How could it not? But it's better that I know when you're feeling like this so I can understand you more." And I meant it.

In our marriage, John wasn't the only one who needed to divulge thoughts he feared would hurt the person he loves most: it also took me a long time to tell him how annoyed I get when he "double checks" if I've used my nebulizer or called my doctor like I said I would. I know his intentions are genuine, but sometimes it's hard enough not being able to carry the laundry or wheezing too much to finish telling a story. I don't need to feel like I also have a built-in babysitter or nurse too. I just want my husband to be a husband and I want to be his wife, not his patient or charge.

I don't want our inevitable frustration and resentment to escalate into depression and anxiety, so we've established the following expectations for each other: he will let me know when he's feeling overwhelmed and we will set aside "illness free" time every week where we each get a break: I don't have to answer questions about how I am feeling, and he doesn't have to hear about the latest research I've uncovered or what debate about PCD I've stumbled across online. Like my parents, we've evolved to the point where we can say "enough is enough" without devastating each another; the challenge now is sustaining that discourse as diseases and complications progress.

On the rare occasions when Jenni's husband admits to feeling overwhelmed or tired of all the demands of illness, she can sympathize. "He's definitely had moments where, rightfully so, he says, 'I'm tired of you not feeling well.' I totally understand that, because I'm tired of it too!" These moments of Steve's surrender are exceedingly rare, so when they do happen, Jenni knows he must really be frustrated. Rather than feel hurt, she tries to look at things from his perspective and understand all the pressure he feels to take care of her, a pressure she considers especially strong in any kind of long-term romantic relationship. Spouses or partners often have this idea that they are supposed to support us in every way, but as Jenni says about her own husband,

"He's a human; he has his limits. It's a challenge, but we try to talk about where we're each coming from."

Facing the fact that chronic illness will never go away entirely can be daunting. Being able to communicate these feelings is important, but having enough social outlets to give each other a break from the particular rigors of caregiving is also an essential part of working through these periods of frustration. Whether it's family members or good friends, having other people who can listen or help you and having other activities and distractions from the constant juggling of multiple roles can ease the pressure on both partners. For example, Jenni has a strong network of people she can call if she wants to talk to someone other than Steve. Inviting friends over to watch movies or help with light housework or cooking are easy ways to remain connected with other people and still get necessary help. It is just as important for healthy spouses to have an outlet; John has weekly racquetball matches and likes to play golf and go rock climbing, activities that do not interest me at all but I am glad he has them.

A fact of chronic illness is that there will always be times when we need help, and there will always be extra responsibilities and burdens on our loved ones as a result. The key is to have enough trust in each other to confront the frustration and take appropriate breaks before the tension becomes unmanageable.

42.

THE CHRONIC INCOME GAP

*Don't underestimate the economic
impact of illness—but don't let
it define you, either*

HEALTH INSURANCE. prescription co-pays. Doctors' visits, diagnostic tests, and hospitalizations. Home care and physical or occupational therapy. Medical supplies and machinery. Even with fairly decent health insurance, John and I pay thousands of dollars in medical expenses out of pocket each year, and my father's monthly health insurance deductible alone is roughly the same cost as a mortgage payment for a five-room condo in one of the most prohibitively expensive real estate markets in the United States.

If you have chronic illness, none of this is new to you. Whether you're an arthritic, a diabetic, a migraine sufferer, an MS patient, or have any other kind of chronic condition, you're familiar with the steady stream of invoices and medical bills that arrive each month, although they might taper off a bit now and again when your condition is stable. In some ways, the economics of illness represent just another minefield of frustration, but given the emotional component of contributing to a household and maintaining an income and a professional identity, it's about so much more than money.

In the debate over health insurance reform, the battle over affordable prescription drugs, and the controversy surrounding the overall state of health care in our country—you know the tension has traction if Michael Moore treats it with the same fervor with which he's approached politics—I worry the "big ticket" aspects of health care economics dwarf all the other inevitable but overlooked implications. The loss of wages due to illness, the more lucrative positions we decline due to our health, the cost of household help or other types of support that are not medically necessary but are necessities nonetheless, all of these factors can put just as much pressure on finances—and by proxy, on relationships—as medical expenditures. Since they are not considerations that are as obvious or immediate as bills and invoices, they can be even more problematic.

When John and I first started discussing our long-term future, I don't think he understood why I immediately worried so much about our finances. After all, planning for the wedding and honeymoon, purchasing a condo, and graduate school were expenses so many couples our ages faced. These weren't what worried me, though. I'd grown up in a household dominated by chronic illness, and I knew firsthand the many ways it saps financial and emotional strength. We were fortunate that in between bouts of disability and serious relapses, my father was successful in his commission-driven industry, but in a sense the fact that we could afford to do all sorts of things to accommodate illness made me even more conscious of just how expensive illness is. There is no way my mother could have worked at any point in the past several years, so if their household depended on two incomes, they'd have been in serious trouble. Physically, neither of them are up to doing yardwork or many of the other little things healthy people take for granted, like bringing Christmas decorations in from the garage. Instead, they have to pay people to do these things, something I think is harder on them emotionally than financially.

"Illness changes everything," my father always said when he had to pay yet another bill, to hire another person to help out, or to eat the cost of prepaid events and vacations that he couldn't take. It was the same thing he said to me when he supplemented my summer wages during my severe CFS flare in high school, when I had to quit a paying internship during college because I was in and out of the hospital too much and he helped me with my rent, when I got walloped with a medical bill that stretched into the thousands my first year in graduate school and he loaned me the money to pay it off so the bill didn't go into collection. He said it to assuage my guilt, to counter the shame and distaste he knew I felt in not being able to pay for these expenses on my own. I wanted nothing more than to be entirely self-sufficient and independent, the very things illness made increasingly difficult at every turn.

In case there are any doubts as to the long-term limitations of illness on finances, consider the following statistic: According to the Centers for Disease Control and the Department of Health and Human Services, the annual economic impact of chronic fatigue syndrome in the United States is $9.1 billion in lost wages and earnings alone, and this does not include medical expenses or disability benefits.[1] If the earnings gap is that staggering for CFS, imagine what it translates into when you factor in all the other chronic and autoimmune disorders. Considering that many diseases like CFS, fibromyalgia, and lupus manifest during prime childbearing and career-building ages, the economic ramifications for younger couples are even more pronounced.

What John first took to be paranoia or excessive anxiety was really my preemptive guilt over lucrative jobs I would have to turn down because I lacked the stamina to do them, and expenses related to being ill, like the hundreds of dollars wasted for trips and dinners and events we had to cancel at the last minute because my health status changed without warning. With all the bills I accrued each month from doctors and drugstores and all the expenses I'd bring into the relationship, I wouldn't be able to earn the income necessary to compensate. I felt guilty about the additional pressure it put on John that we wouldn't be able to rely on my income or benefits if it ever came to that. Intellectually, I knew he realized we would have lots of medical bills and health care costs, but I worried he didn't realize how deeply illness would penetrate into our financial flexibility and choices. He grew up in a quintessentially healthy household; even in their mid- to late fifties, his parents can still spend whole weekend days outside mowing their beautiful lawn, cutting down trees, and transplanting bushes.

How could I account for the inevitable economic realities of illness without completely defining our relationship and our financial potential through them? How can any of us resolve that?

My guilt was mixed with the fear that John would start to resent the way my illnesses limited his financial choices too. We were tested within months of our wedding when his company was sold and the entire workforce was laid off. Unemployment and looking for a new job is stressful no matter what, but when your wife is chronically ill and depends on expensive medications and daily physical therapy to stay out of the hospital, the pressure is omnipresent. I can't help but think back to Rosalind Joffe's comments about chronically ill people needing to make less-than-ideal career trajectory choices if it means finding a job in a company with more flexible attitudes or values. In a sense, the same kind of restricted options are sometimes part of healthy spouses' decision making as well. John had specific requirements for his next job in terms of his long-term career goals, but some of them had to be pushed aside because at the end of the day, we needed a steady paycheck and health insurance. The immediate demands of my health problems subsumed his ability to be as selective and strategic as he'd have like to have been.

I'd been so focused on all the ways my problems would impact us collectively that I hadn't even teased out the very personal ways it would affect John until we were confronted with his unemployment. I could feel guilty about that and compound the already volatile flux of guilt and overcompensation I was experiencing, or I could look at it this way: I had a husband who was willing to be flexible with his needs and desires for my benefit. I owed it to him to be grateful, not guilty. *Illness changes everything.* I had thought since I was the one with all the experience with illness that I had everything to teach John; instead, I had a lot of learning to do too.

43.

"CAN" VERSUS "SHOULD":
THE BABY GAME

Weighing medicine's odds with
individual circumstances is not easy,
but it is imperative

I N THIS DAY AND AGE, I can get almost anyone pregnant," my fertility specialist said. "Of course, the real
question is, just because someone can get pregnant, *should*
that someone get pregnant?"

It wasn't a hypothetical question; she'd just told me that
because of my PCD I had a 75 percent chance of not being
able to have children on my own. Like the cilia in the respiratory system, the cilia in the reproductive system often do
not work, and the fallopian tubes need healthy cilia to move
fertilized eggs.

Of all the questions debated in medicine today, "can versus should" is one of the most significant, one with the
power to reshape our thinking about serious chronic illness
and the advancements of medical technology. It was the

question many couples with all kinds of chronic illnesses grapple with this in their bedrooms and their doctors' offices every day, the same one John and I had been circling around for months. Pregnancy and childbirth are inherently risky; after all, healthy people encounter complications and unexpected obstacles all the time. Knowing this, knowing all the variables stacked against us, and knowing that women with PCD have carried and delivered healthy babies, what was our answer going to be?

Before we'd gotten engaged—actually, before we'd even discussed the idea of marriage—John had taken me aback by announcing one night over margaritas that if we were ever to get married and having children came down to me putting my health or life in danger, he would adopt children in a heartbeat.

"I'm not someone who would get hung up on wanting a biological child to keep my genes going. I want you to be healthy and I'd never want you to feel you needed to put yourself at risk," he said.

We hadn't even discussed having children together, let alone getting married, so his bringing the topic up made me aware of how serious he was about our future.

Between the two of us, we have five nieces and we adore them. We volunteer to babysit to get time alone with them, and our refrigerator and all available coffee table and shelf space is covered with their pictures: two little girls hugging their dog at Christmas, the newest baby in her Easter bonnet, a toddler on her second birthday, trying to fit a huge cookie into her mouth all at once. In white and lilac satin dresses with big bows and wreaths in their hair, two of them were flower girls at our wedding, and our oldest niece did one of the readings during the nuptial Mass, instantly winning over the church crowd with her sweet young voice and precise pronunciation. Throughout our engagement, relatives at family parties would elbow each other and point toward the two of us and whichever niece we were playing with and smile knowingly, as if to say "You two look ready for kids of your own soon." Sometimes they said as much to us, and we brushed it off in that half-embarrassed, half-pleased way.

After the fertility consult we had an in-depth consult with a doctor from high-risk fetal medicine, whose total honesty and thorough analysis of the "can versus should" scenario only tangled us up further with questions and deliberations. In fact, the more we looked at the situation, the more questions we realized we might never get concrete answers to—and yet these imprecise estimates and guesses were all we had at our disposal when making such life-altering decisions. Luckily we did know that women with PCD have delivered healthy babies, and that was the most important thing. The fact PCD is a rare disease and there is limited data available on PCD and pregnancy made it more difficult to tease out options, and there are lots of women out there with rare diseases facing the same lack of pregnancy-related information. I could glean some of the pregnancy-related risks I would face from the similar situations CF and other respiratory patients encountered, but in terms of actually conceiving children, there is only so much medicine could tell me. In fact, other than trying indefinitely and never getting pregnant, the only "true" way we'd know if the cilia in my fallopian tubes were defective would be if I had an ectopic pregnancy, where the fertilized egg develops outside the uterus, usually in the fallopian tubes. Without proper room to grow, the embryo typically bursts, causing severe bleeding and sometimes putting the mother's life at risk.

"That's kind of a lousy way to find out for sure, huh?" I said to John, trying to pass it off as another "just my luck" moment, when in reality we were both chastened by the news. Our specialist gave us a sympathetic look.

The particular risks for pregnant women with chronic conditions are obviously dependent on the nature of the illness. For me, between compromised oxygenation for the fetus and the threat of severe infection, as well as the risks of certain medications used to treat the infections, we learned the highest risk for us, as it is for many, would be preterm labor. The doctor guided us through the differences in outcomes for babies born at twenty-four weeks compared with those born at twenty-eight weeks, thirty-two weeks, and higher. She wanted to make sure we understood the consequences of giving birth to a baby at each of these stages. The point where it becomes healthier for a preterm baby to fight for life outside the womb rather than inside varies from woman to woman, and it is difficult to know what a woman's threshold will be until she hits it and it is time to act.

This was the conversation Vicki and Dan had with her doctors when they first discussed having children. In fact, their conversations were even more stark given that Vicki's health had already deteriorated significantly by the time she was in her early thirties and ready to have children. Her lung function was well below the minimum level recommended for pregnancy and the only way her physician would condone her to consider carrying her own child was if she agreed to the following stipulations: no breastfeeding since she couldn't spare the calories; she had to have live-in help so she'd have the energy to care for her child; and she could only deliver one child.

"I wanted my child more than anything, but I really suffered. I'd do it again in a heartbeat, but I was prepared from day one to sacrifice my life for my child," she says. There's no doubt her pregnancy caused her health to decline even further; she was hospitalized several times when she couldn't breathe and get enough air, and she lost weight just when her body needed to gain it the most. Though it was grueling and fraught with complications, Vicki held on until she reached thirty-four weeks, when her son was born. Fortunately, her son had no long-term health complications from premature birth and is now a healthy toddler.

"When I look at my son, I feel a love like I've never experienced before. I've never wanted to be so close to someone in my life. He's the best Prozac, the best sun on a rainy day," she says. Still, the realities of her chronic condition are not entirely muted by her joy, realities so many patients who live into adulthood with serious illnesses and consider having children must face. She gets frustrated when she needs her husband or her nanny's help caring for her son, and there are many nights when she is awake, restless at the thought that something could happen to her.

"I can't imagine my son growing up without me, but it's something my husband and I have talked about. It's torture to think of leaving him. Talk about control issues," she says. For Vicki, the pros clearly outweigh the cons of motherhood, but there are days when she wishes she could focus exclusively on her son and not have to deal with all these scenarios that healthy parents do not have to consider.

For as dogged as she was to have a child, Vicki was equally prepared and pragmatic about it. Every decision she and Dan made, from the decision not to use a surrogate to carry their child or look into adoption to which nanny to hire, was preceded by copious amounts of research and evaluation of potential consequences. She knew surrogacy wasn't right for her personality, and she also worried that her disease status would prevent her and Dan from being able to adopt a child. Luckily, Vicki conceived her son within a few months and did not have to start assisted reproductive techniques, but she knows if she wants any more children, she will not be able to carry them on her own.

Like many prospective parents with inheritable diseases in their personal or family history, they made sure Dan was tested to see if he carried the CF gene before they tried to conceive; his results were negative. Because of their Jewish heritage, their genetic counselor also recommended they both be tested for Tay-Sachs disease, a fatal genetic disorder whose incidence is higher in people of Jewish descent. The genetic profiles for couples considering pregnancy obviously differ depending on the types of inheritable diseases involved and the ability to isolate the mutations that cause them, but speaking with a genetic counselor can help potential parents who are worried about passing on diseases navigate this complicated situation and assess their risks.

Vicki's experience also yields another compelling (and equally complicated) component of the can-versus-should scenario: socioeconomics. She had to agree to constant help in order for her doctors to support her pregnancy. What if that option was not feasible financially?

"If we couldn't afford a nanny or day care and had no scheduled or committed help from family or friends on a daily basis, I probably couldn't have had my son. I was pretty sick before I got pregnant. I physically couldn't care for him," she says. She had been warned that the hardest part of having a baby would come after the delivery, but until she was home with her son and struggling to muster the energy to care for him, she didn't really understand the truth of that statement. Because of how sick she is, she feels it would have been selfish to ask her husband and her family and everyone involved in her well-being who have already done so much for her to step in and assume care for her child if she couldn't afford help.

"There are no easy answers," she admits. "I've made important decisions in my life, like who I married, a man I knew could make a good living, and where I live—around the corner from my mom, who can help me—so that I am better able to get all I want out of life. I've tried to position myself in the best way possible for my future," she says, hitting at the core of what every patient contemplating having children needs to decide. What does that ideal position look like, and what do we need to do to get there? The answer is as varied and idiosyncratic as the patients and diseases involved, but the essence remains the same.

Vicki's story lends both incredible hope and invaluable insights to all of us considering children, regardless of our particular medical conditions and complications. It brings to focus those many questions we need to be asking: Are you in a financially feasible situation to stop working early in the pregnancy, if it comes to that? Will you be able to procure help if your health deteriorates and you need it, and if not, who will cover the gaps? If you can't have children on your own, how do you want to proceed? Are you prepared emotionally and financially for the spectrum of outcomes that accompany a high-risk pregnancy? And lastly, as our fertility specialist and the high-risk obstetrician gingerly but deliberately hinted at, are you prepared to draw a firm line about how far you are willing to go with fertility treatments before you consider adoption or surrogacy?

Even though she is only twenty and is still in college, Jade is already thinking about whether or not to have children. Inheritability is paramount among her concerns; if future genetic testing reveals she could pass on her condition to her child, she is not comfortable with the idea of giving her son or daughter a potential lifetime of pain. She also has serious worries about the more pragmatic aspects of carrying a child. When she has a severe pain flare, it is her back and abdomen that hurt, the areas of the body pregnancy strains anyway. The pain is excruciating enough on its own; she can't imagine how much worse it would be if she experienced a severe flare while pregnant, especially if she were unable to take strong pain medication.

But her biggest concern is whether she can provide the kind of care and attention she wants for her children. "I can barely take care of myself when the pain is really bad, never mind my baby," she says. If Jade were ever in a situation where there was no one else to depend on for help, she just doesn't think she could manage being a single parent with a serious medical condition. It wouldn't be fair to place her child in a position where he or she wasn't getting the time, attention, and resources children need. These aren't questions she can answer definitively, but they are ones she knows she needs to be honest about as she moves forward.

Jade and Vicki both touch on one of the biggest obstacles women with all types of chronic or debilitating conditions face: the "bad days" we experience become much worse when they impact our ability to care for our children. The intensity and frequency of bad days vary from woman to woman, disease to disease. For women with less serious conditions or whose flares aren't completely incapacitating, the circumstances are a little bit different and the extenuating economic and logistical factors may not be as pronounced. In Vicki's case, the severity of her CF necessitated the degree of restrictions and contingency plans she, Dan, and her medical team agreed on for her pregnancy and child care.

Being realistic about the demands of child care as well as your disease progression is vital when you are trying to map the best plan for you and your family. In addition to detailed discussions with physicians, connecting with patients who have the same conditions and have already gone through pregnancy or infertility is an important way to assess your situation. Thinking back to the concept of community health discussed previously, I can't imagine a more suitable application for the shared patient experience. For so many women, this is fairly new medical territory, and sometimes that patient narrative that is so fundamental to medicine is equally valuable from a patient-to-patient perspective.

Some of these issues—infertility, child care, economics—are certainly ones plenty of women who are otherwise healthy face. I'm not implying they are exclusive to chronic illness; it's just that the same conversations are that much more thorny when illness is part of the dialogue.

"I can't give you any odds about any of the complications we've discussed. You'll get sicker more often than you do now and you will take longer to recover. You will spend more time in the hospital than you do now and you have to be prepared for the fact you might not be able to work for most of your pregnancy," our fetal medicine physician told us at the end of our exhaustive consult. I swallowed the lump in my throat and stole a sideways glance at John.

"But if anyone with your particular constellation of complex problems has a chance at a favorable outcome, I would say it's you," she added.

At last, a glimmer of optimism cut through the staggering list of possibilities and questions.

"You're educated, informed, and a proactive patient. In that sense, you're ideal," she said. I dared to smile at her.

When John and I sat down in a coffee shop to digest all that had been said at our consult, we clung to her parting words. I might not end up in that 25 percent of women with PCD who can have children on their own, and we might not get the types of ratios and percents we'd like as we move forward, but we'll deal with that if need be. I've always hated being defined by numbers—how many conditions, how many surgeries, how many medications—and my doctor's words reminded me that I cannot add up all those parts and get a whole me. It's important to remember that none of us with chronic illness should start speaking the language of numbers exclusively, since they will always fail to capture what is the most important element: hope.

44.

HOMEOSTASIS

*Being well has nothing to do with
being healthy*

HOMEOSTASIS. I'VE ALWAYS LATCHED onto that word, intrigued by the concept of the body's internal point of equilibrium, the place where the hormones and the mechanisms and the things taken in and things expelled are balanced. I doubted my body would ever maintain homeostasis, but I assumed that was because of all of my chronic conditions. Only recently have I realized that I cannot compartmentalize the physical and the emotional any more than I can separate symptoms of certain conditions from the side effects of others—they morph into one another in such a way that the point of origin is no longer distinguishable or significant. True homeostasis has little to do with the scientific term and everything to do with balancing the competing needs of the body and the spirit. I was so accustomed to illness throwing my life into chaos that I lived in a state of perpetual alertness—except that in waiting so vigilantly for illness to change things for me, I didn't let myself see that perhaps I had finally made the kinds of decisions that would better allow me to live *with* illness, not in spite of it.

My moment of truth came the fall after our wedding, when I had the confidence to begin writing about my health publicly for the first time. The night before my personal essay on chronic illness and dating appeared in the *Boston Globe Magazine*, I was anxious about how much of my private life I was revealing, but I was also relieved. I wrote what I knew, and what I knew after all these years was that the only way chronic illness can overwhelm a relationship is if you allow it to—and while I wrote in reference to romantic relationships, I knew it applied to every other kind of relationship too. For me to bring my conditions and my fears about them to a mainstream reading audience was proof to myself that I had found my personal homeostasis—my life wasn't segmented into the roles of patient, writer, teacher, wife, friend, daughter, aunt. It was a fluid combination of all of them. I'd struggled for years with the idea of balancing the private, inner world of illness and the public, external world of the healthy. I was tired of fighting my innate urge to ignore illness, to prove I could be defined by any amount of superlatives or roles *except* that of patient.

Illness has always been a part of my life, just as it has been for so many patients and all the people we choose to bring into our lives. It always will. Admitting this doesn't mean resignation, but release. It's a process of first accepting the realities of our conditions and then integrating them into our perceptions of ourselves. I remember the first time John ever told me he sometimes forgot I was even sick. We were sitting on my couch in Beacon Hill, my last apartment as a single girl, and laughing. I don't remember what exactly we found so funny, but I know I laughed so hard that I started to cough. I coughed for a few minutes, then jumped up and sprinted to the bathroom just in time to cough up some phlegm. I returned to the couch and tried to pick up the conversation where we had left off, but John's eyes were narrowed in concern, even a hint of sadness. When I probed, he answered, "It just hit me, is all. We were just sitting here and then you were coughing so hard, and I forgot how easy it is for things to change, because I don't always remember you're sick."

What he said was one of the best things he could have done for me, because he allowed me to see myself as he saw me. I was the woman he loved who happened to be sick; I wasn't the sick woman he loved. It was as easy as that.

There is no doubt illness brings definition to our lives—of the many commonalities among the stories from patients I've collected in this book, that is the most pervasive. I think about Vicki's son or Jenni's expanding business, and I consider how the experience of being a patient has influenced these roles. I think about Brian's career plans, Kerri's diabetic column, Jade's plans for after she graduates, or Angela's desire to get her degree and pursue medical school despite her EDS, and I see the ways illness has inserted itself into their decisions—it is present, it is something that demands accommodation, but it is not the ultimate indicator of who they are or what their potential is.

Our various stories are at once both specific and collective of the basic experience of living with any illness. In the end, symptoms and treatments aside, we all know that illness pushes us and we push back and that somewhere along the way, we figure out how to rebound with falling too far on either side. That place where we stand on even ground, neither shoving back too hard nor falling too low, represents what it means to be well.

And being well, it turns out, has nothing to do with being healthy.

ACKNOWLEDGMENTS

The ongoing guidance and foresight of my wonderful agent, Matthew Carnicelli, turned this book from a mere possibility into a reality. My publisher, George Gibson, believed in this project from the first page of the proposal and has been outspoken in his enthusiasm ever since. Jackie Johnson, my editor, recognized at once that there was an audience that needed to be reached by this book and has nurtured its development at every turn. The entire team at Walker & Company has given my book the perfect home, and their hard work and dedication have been instrumental to its development.

This project would never have made it across an agent's desk without the help of my professors and fellow writers in Emerson College's MFA program. I am grateful for the constructive criticism and encouragement of Joseph Hurka, Pamela Painter, and especially Douglas Whynott, whose nonfiction writing workshop gave me the space to become a more focused writer and a more critical reader. Lissa Warren's class on book publicity was an indispensable tool. My cousin Alice Sapienza is my mentor and signpost in all things related to writing and is a thoughtful reader of everything I write. The lovely ladies of SWiG have made me a part of their amazing writing group and have given me invaluable feedback throughout the draft stages.

The candor and insights of the patients interviewed in this book—Angela Ayoub, Jade Cooper, Vicki Klein, Kerri Morrone, Jenni Prokopy, and Brian Sercus—are a source of inspiration and much appreciation on my part. Jenni has been a champion of my writing even before there was a book, and first connected me with the brilliant medblogging community. This book is also much richer due to the expertise and perspective of Richard Anderson, Rosalind Joffe, Paula Kravitz, and Lynn Royster.

Any clarity or wisdom about the doctor-patient relationship I may have accumulated over the years is largely due to the dedicated physicians who have made a huge difference in my life. Dr. Marvin Fried, Dr. Henry Dorkin, and Dr. Bruce Levy are among the best of the best. Steve Jurkowski is not only a top-notch physical therapist; he's also a true friend and a wonderful listener.

I am blessed to have loyal friends who have stood by me through the many ups and downs of my illnesses and have found the humor in every unbelievable situation. Nicole Langan's friendship has spanned decades. Catherine Camm, Meghann Ward, Jason Wuliger, Betsy Verrill, Tina Shaughnessy, Caitlin Connelly, Frosina Panovska, Michelle Melka, Laura Dicker, and many others have been true friends— from long-distance calls and hospital sleepovers to home visits and chest PT, they have given me much to write about.

None of this would have been possible without the emotional and oftentimes physical support of my family. My brothers, Marc and Michael, have always been incredibly compassionate and supportive of me. My father, the most determined, generous, and optimistic person I know, has shown me the measure of a true hero. My mother is my biggest advocate. Her tireless encouragement and unconditional love give me strength when I need it and inspiration when I seek it.

Lastly, my husband, John, read every draft of every chapter in this book. In addition to being a diligent and thoughtful editor, he has been unwavering in his belief in me. He is as caring as he is patient, he is as intuitive as he is intelligent, and I am a better person and better writer for having him in my life.

APPENDIX OF ADDITIONAL RESOURCES

Employment

Americans with Disabilities Act
http://www.usdoj.gov/crt/ada/adahom1.htm

Chronic Illness Coach: Resource for Professionals Living with Chronic Illness
http://cicoach.com

Job Accommodation Network (a free service of the U.S. Department of Labor)
http://www.jan.wvu.edu

U.S. Department of Labor, Office of Disability Employment Policy
http://www.dol.gov/odep

U.S. Equal Employment Opportunity Commission
http://www.eeoc.gov

Education

American College Health Association
http://www.acha.org

Center for Young Women's Health, "Impact of Chronic Illness on College Planning"
http://www.youngwomenshealth.org/impact.html

The Chronic Illness Initiative, DePaul University
http://www.snl.depaul.edu/current/chronic.asp

Health Insurance and Advocacy

Advocacy for Patients with Chronic Illness
http://www.advocacyforpatients.org

Center for Medical Consumers
http://www.medicalconsumers.org

Every Patient's Advocate
http://www.everypatientsadvocate.com

Families USA: The Voice for Health Care Consumers
http://www.familiesusa.org

HealthInsuranceInfo.net, Georgetown University Health Policy Institute
http://www.healthinsuranceinfo.net

National Council for Support of Disability Issues
http://www.ncsd.org

National Women's Health Network
http://nwhn.org

NeedyMeds: Information You Need to Get Your Medicine
http://www.needymeds.com

Patient Advocate Foundation
http://www.patientadvocate.org

Patients Are Powerful
http://www.patientsarepowerful.org

Social Security and Disability Resource Center
http://www.ssdrc.com

General Chronic Illness

American Autoimmune Related Diseases Association
http://www.aarda.org

American Chronic Pain Association
http://www.theacpa.org

American Pain Foundation
http://www.painfoundation.org

But You Don't Look Sick?
http://www.butyoudontlooksick.com

ChronicBabe (an online community for younger women with health issues)
http://www.chronicbabe.com

HealingWell.com: A Guide to Diseases, Disorders, and Chronic Illness
http://www.healingwell.com

How to Cope with Pain
http://www.howtocopewithpain.org

Improving Chronic Illness Care
http://www.improvingchroniccare.org

Invisible Disabilities Advocate
http://www.myida.org

National Foundation for the Treatment of Pain
http://www.paincare.org

National Organization for Rare Disorders
http://www.rarediseases.org

For Families and Caregivers

Family Caregiver Alliance
http://www.caregiver.org/caregiver/jsp/home.jsp

Moms in Flight (for mothers with chronic illness)
http://www.momsinflight.bravepages.com

National Family Caregivers Association
http://www.nfcacares.org

Sibling Support Project (for brothers and sisters of people who
have special health, developmental, or mental health concerns)
http://www.siblingsupport.org

Well Spouse Association
http://www.wellspouse.org

For Teens

C. Everett Koop Institute: Chronic Illness Resources for Teens
http://dms.dartmouth.edu/koop/resources/chronic_illness

GirlsHealth.gov: Illness and Disability
http://www.girlshealth.gov/disability/index.htm

(All urls valid as of November 9, 2007)

NOTES

CHAPTER 1

1. David B. Morris, *Illness and Culture in the Postmodern Age* (Berkeley: University of California Press, 2000), 36–37.

CHAPTER 2

1. Jerome Groopman, MD, *How Doctors Think* (Boston: Houghton Mifflin, 2007), 24.

2. Ibid., 5.

CHAPTER 3

1. Celiac Sprue Association, "Celiac Disease Defined," *http://csaceliacs.org/celiac_defined.php* (accessed May 2, 2007).

CHAPTER 18

1. National Organization of Rare Disorders "About NORD," http://www.rarediseases.org/info/about.html (accessed June 8, 2007).

CHAPTER 19

1. "Culture Clash: Kids with Chronic Illness Face Difficult Transition to Adult Care," *University of Florida News*, February 23, 2005, *http://news.ufl.edu/2005/02/23/docswap* (accessed May 18, 2007).

2. DePaul University, "The Chronic Illness Initiative," *http://www.snl.depaul.edu/current/chronic.asp* (accessed February 19, 2007).

CHAPTER 22

1. Kevin T. Stroupe, Eleanor D. Kinney, and Thomas J. J. Kniesner, "Chronic Illness and Health Insurance-Related Job Lock." *Journal of Policy Analysis and Management* 20, no. 3 (2001), 525.

2. Ibid.

CHAPTER 24

1. PBS, "Who Cares: Chronic Illness in America," *http://www.pbs.org/inthebalance/archives/whocares/awareness/what_is.html* (accessed May 26, 2007).

CHAPTER 28

1. Jean Ashton, "Life After the Shock! The Impact on Families of Caring for Young Children with Chronic Illness," *Australian Journal of Early Childhood* 29: 1 (March 2004), 26.

CHAPTER 29

1. Donald Sharpe and Lucille Rossiter, "Siblings of Children with a Chronic Illness: A Meta-Analysis," *Journal of Pediatric Psychology* 27, no. 8 (2002), 706.

CHAPTER 40

1. Rest Ministries, "National Invisible Chronic Illness Week," *http://www.mychronicillness.com/invisibleillness/statistics.htm* (accessed June 15, 2007).

2. Phyllis A. Gordon and Kristin M. Perrone, "When Spouses Become Caregivers: Counseling Implications for Younger Couples," *Journal of Rehabilitation* 70, no. 2 (April–June 2004), 27.

3. Ibid.

4. Ibid., 31.

CHAPTER 41

1. Phyllis A. Gordon and Kristin M. Perrone, "When Spouses Become Caregivers: Counseling Implications for Younger Couples," *Journal of Rehabilitation* 70, no. 2 (April–June 2004), 27.

2. Ibid.

CHAPTER 42

1. Centers for Disease Control and Prevention, "Chronic Fatigue Syndrome: Missions/Goals," http://www.cdc.gov/cfs/mission.htm (accessed November 27, 2007).

INDEX

ABOUT THE AUTHOR

Laurie Edwards is a health journalist whose essays and articles have been published in the *Boston Globe* and on several online sites, including ChronicBabe.com. Her blog, A Chronic Dose (www.AChronicDose.com), was named one the top-10 sites for chronic pain by the Health Central Network. Despite having several chronic illnesses, Edwards received an undergraduate degree from Georgetown University and MFA in creative writing from Emerson College and teaches writing at Northeastern University. This is her first book. She lives with her husband in Boston, Massachusetts.